Socioeconomics of Neuroimaging

Guest Editor

DAVID M. YOUSEM, MD, MBA

NEUROIMAGING CLINICS OF NORTH AMERICA

www.neuroimaging.theclinics.com

Consulting Editor
SURESH K. MUKHERJI, MD

August 2012 • Volume 22 • Number 3

SAUNDERS an imprint of ELSEVIER, Inc.

W.B. SAUNDERS COMPANY
A Division of Elsevier Inc.

1600 John F. Kennedy Boulevard • Suite 1800 • Philadelphia, Pennsylvania 19103-2899

http://www.theclinics.com

NEUROIMAGING CLINICS OF NORTH AMERICA Volume 22, Number 3
August 2012 ISSN 1052-5149, ISBN 13: 978-1-4557-4885-3

Editor: Sarah E. Barth
Developmental Editor: Donald Mumford

Neuroimaging Clinics of North America (ISSN 1052-5149) is published quarterly by Elsevier Inc., 360 Park Avenue South, New York, NY 10010-1710. Months of issue are February, May, August, and November. Business and editorial offices: 1600 John F. Kennedy Blvd., Suite 1800, Philadelphia, PA 19103-2899. Business and editorial offices: 6277 Sea Harbor Drive, Orlando, FL 32887-4800. Periodicals postage paid at New York, NY, and additional mailing offices. Subscription prices are USD 342 per year for US individuals, USD 471 per year for US institutions, USD 172 per year for US students and residents, USD 396 per year for Canadian individuals, USD 590 per year for Canadian institutions, USD 502 per year for international individuals, USD 590 per year for international institutions and USD 246 per year for Canadian and foreign students and residents. To receive student/resident rate, orders must be accompanied by name of affiliated institution, date of term, and the *signature* of program/residency coordinator on institution letterhead. Orders will be billed at individual rate until proof of status is received. Foreign air speed delivery is included in all *Clinics* subscription prices. All prices are subject to change without notice. POSTMASTER: Send address changes to *Neuroimaging Clinics of North America*, Elsevier Health Sciences Division, Subscription Customer Service, 3251 Riverport Lane, Maryland Heights, MO 63043. Telephone: 1-800-654-2452 (U.S. and Canada); 314-447-8871 (outside U.S. and Canada). Fax: 314-447-8029. E-mail: journalscustomerservice-usa@elsevier.com (for print support); journalsonlinesupport-usa@elsevier.com (for online support).

Reprints. For copies of 100 or more of articles in this publication, please contact the Commercial Reprints Department, Elsevier Inc., 360 Park Avenue South, New York, NY 10010-1710. Tel.: 212-633-3812; Fax: 212-462-1935; E-mail: reprints@elsevier.com.

Neuroimaging Clinics of North America is covered by *Excerpta Medical/EMBASE,* the RSNA Index of Imaging Literature, *MEDLINE/PubMed (Index Medicus),* MEDLINE/MEDLARS, SciSearch, Research Alert, and Neuroscience Citation Index.

Printed and bound by CPI Group (UK) Ltd, Croydon, CR0 4YY

Transferred to Digital Print 2012

GOAL STATEMENT

The goal of *Neuroimaging Clinics of North America* is to keep practicing radiologists and radiology residents up to date with current clinical practice in radiology by providing timely articles reviewing the state of the art in patient care.

ACCREDITATION

The *Neuroimaging Clinics of North America* is planned and implemented in accordance with the Essential Areas and Policies of the Accreditation Council for Continuing Medical Education (ACCME) through the joint sponsorship of the University of Virginia School of Medicine and Elsevier. The University of Virginia School of Medicine is accredited by the ACCME to provide continuing medical education for physicians.

The University of Virginia School of Medicine designates this enduring material activity for a maximum of 15 *AMA PRA Category 1 Credit*(s)™ for each issue, 60 credits per year. Physicians should claim only the credit commensurate with the extent of their participation in the activity.

The American Medical Association has determined that physicians not licensed in the US who participate in this CME enduring material activity are eligible for a maximum of 15 *AMA PRA Category 1 Credit*(s)™ for each issue, 60 credits per year.

Credit can be earned by reading the text material, taking the CME examination online at http://www.theclinics.com/home/cme, and completing the evaluation. After taking the test, you will be required to review any and all incorrect answers. Following completion of the test and evaluation, your credit will be awarded and you may print your certificate.

FACULTY DISCLOSURE/CONFLICT OF INTEREST

The University of Virginia School of Medicine, as an ACCME accredited provider, endorses and strives to comply with the Accreditation Council for Continuing Medical Education (ACCME) Standards of Commercial Support, Commonwealth of Virginia statutes, University of Virginia policies and procedures, and associated federal and private regulations and guidelines on the need for disclosure and monitoring of proprietary and financial interests that may affect the scientific integrity and balance of content delivered in continuing medical education activities under our auspices.

The University of Virginia School of Medicine requires that all CME activities accredited through this institution be developed independently and be scientifically rigorous, balanced and objective in the presentation/discussion of its content, theories and practices.

All authors/editors participating in an accredited CME activity are expected to disclose to the readers relevant financial relationships with commercial entities occurring within the past 12 months (such as grants or research support, employee, consultant, stock holder, member of speakers bureau, etc.). The University of Virginia School of Medicine will employ appropriate mechanisms to resolve potential conflicts of interest to maintain the standards of fair and balanced education to the reader. Questions about specific strategies can be directed to the Office of Continuing Medical Education, University of Virginia School of Medicine, Charlottesville, Virginia.

The faculty and staff of the University of Virginia Office of Continuing Medical Education have no financial affiliations to disclose.

The authors/editors listed below have identified no professional/financial affiliations for themselves or their spouse/partner:

Nikesh Anumula, MD; Sarah Barth, (Acquisitions Editor); Jacqueline Bello, MD; William D. Donovan, MD, MPH; Adam E. Flanders, MD; Paul E. Kim, MD; Paras Lakhani, MD; Frank J. Lexa, MD, MBA; Indu R. Meesa, MD, MS; Govind Mukundan, MD; Francisco A. Perez, MD, PhD; Pina C. Sanelli, MD, MPH; Lubdha M. Shah, MD (Test Author); and David M. Youssem, MD, MBA (Guest Editor).

The authors listed below have identified the following professional/financial affiliations for themselves or their spouse/partner:

Jonathan W. Berlin, MD, MBA is on the Advisory Board and is a stockholder for Nuance Communications.
William G. Bradley Jr, MD, PhD is an industry funded research/investigator for GE.
Jeffrey G. Jarvik, MD, MPH is on the Advisory/Committee Board for GE Healthcare; is a consultant for HealthHelp; has stock/ownership and is a patent holder for PysioSonics; was a one time speaker at a Synthes sponsored course.
Robert A. Meeker, MA, MS is employed by Spectrum Health.
Suresh K. Mukherji, MD (Consulting Editor) is a consultant for Philips.
David Seidenwurm, MD is employed by and has stock in Radiological Assoc. of SAC; also employed by and on the speakers bureau for ACR; is an industry funded research/investigator and on the advisory committee board with stock in Aaken Labs; is a consultant for BCBS Cancer Center Program.
Mark S. Shiroishi, MD is a consultant for Bayer, and receives research support from GE Healthcare.
Patrick A. Turski, MD is an industry funded research/investigator for GE Healthcare, and owns stock in Ultasonix.

Disclosure of Discussion of Non-FDA Approved Uses for Pharmaceutical Products and/or Medical Devices.

The University of Virginia School of Medicine, as an ACCME provider, requires that all faculty presenters identify and disclose any off-label uses for pharmaceutical and medical device products. The University of Virginia School of Medicine recommends that each physician fully review all the available data on new products or procedures prior to clinical use.

TO ENROLL

To enroll in the Neuroimaging Clinics of North America Continuing Medical Education program, call customer service at 1-800-654-2452 or sign up online at http://www.theclinics.com/home/cme. The CME program is available to subscribers for an additional annual fee of USD 196.

NEUROIMAGING CLINICS OF NORTH AMERICA

FORTHCOMING ISSUES

Intracranial Infections
Gaurang Shah, MD, *Guest Editor*

Pediatric Demyelinating Disease and its Mimics
Manohar Shroff, MD, *Guest Editor*

MR Spectroscopy
Lara Brandão, MD, *Guest Editor*

MR Neurography
Avneesh Chhabra, MD, *Guest Editor*

RECENT ISSUES

May 2012
Neuroradiology Applications of High-Field MR Imaging
Winfried A. Willinek, MD, *Guest Editor*

February 2012
Imaging in Alzheimer's Disease and Other Dementias
Alison D. Murray, MBChB (Hons), FRCP, FRCR, *Guest Editor*

November 2011
Neuroimaging of Tropical Disease
Rakesh K. Gupta, MD, *Guest Editor*

RELATED INTEREST

Radiologic Clinics, Vol. 50, No. 4, July 2012
Spine Imaging
Timothy P. Maus, MD, *Guest Editor*

Contributors

CONSULTING EDITOR

SURESH K. MUKHERJI, MD, FACR
Director of Neuroradiology, Professor and
Chief of Neuroradiology and Head & Neck
Radiology; Professor of Radiology,
Otolaryngology Head Neck Surgery, Radiation
Oncology, Periodontics and Oral Medicine,
University of Michigan Health System,
Ann Arbor, Michigan

GUEST EDITOR

DAVID M. YOUSEM, MD, MBA
Professor of Radiology, Director of
Neuroradiology, Vice Chairman of Program
Development, Associate Dean of Professional
Development, Russell H. Morgan Department
of Radiology and Radiological Sciences, Johns
Hopkins Medical Institution, Baltimore,
Maryland

AUTHORS

NIKESH ANUMULA, MD
Department of Radiology, Weill Cornell
Medical College, New York-Presbyterian
Hospital, New York, New York

JACQUELINE BELLO, MD
Professor of Clinical Radiology and
Neurosurgery, Director of Neuroradiology,
Montefiore Medical Center, Albert Einstein
College of Medicine, New York, New York

JONATHAN W. BERLIN, MD, MBA
Clinical Associate Professor of Radiology,
NorthShore University HealthSystem,
University of Chicago Pritzker School of
Medicine, Evanston, Illinois

WILLIAM G. BRADLEY Jr, MD, PhD, FACR
Professor and Chairman, Department of
Radiology, UCSD Medical Center, San Diego,
California

WILLIAM D. DONOVAN, MD, MPH, FACR
Department of Diagnostic Imaging, The William
W. Backus Hospital, Norwich, Connecticut

ADAM E. FLANDERS, MD
Professor of Radiology and Rehabilitation
Medicine, Department of Radiology, Division of
Neuroradiology/ENT, Thomas Jefferson
University Hospital, Philadelphia, Pennsylvania

JEFFREY G. JARVIK, MD, MPH
Professor of Radiology and Neurological
Surgery, Department of Radiology, Harborview
Medical Center, School of Medicine; Director,
Comparative Effectiveness, Cost and
Outcomes Research Center; Department of
Neurological Surgery, School of Medicine;
Adjunct Professor of Health Services and
Pharmacy, Department of Health Services,
School of Public Health, University of
Washington, Seattle, Washington

PAUL E. KIM, MD
Assistant Professor of Clinical Radiology,
University of Southern California Keck School
of Medicine, Los Angeles, California

PARAS LAKHANI, MD
Department of Radiology, Thomas Jefferson
University Hospital, Philadelphia, Pennsylvania

FRANK J. LEXA, MD, MBA
Vice Chairman and Professor of Radiology,
Drexel University College of Medicine, and
Adjunct Professor of Marketing, Project Faculty,
Spain, United Arab Emirates and East Asia
Regional Manager, Global Consulting Practicum,
The Wharton School, Philadelphia, Pennsylvania;
Professor of Business Development in the Life
Sciences, Instituto de Empresa, Madrid, Spain

ROBERT A. MEEKER, MA, MS
Strategic Program Manager, Administration,
Spectrum Health Hospitals, Grand Rapids,
Michigan

INDU REKHA MEESA, MD, MS
Diagnostic Radiology Resident, Grand Rapids
Medical Education Partners; Michigan State
University, Spectrum Health Hospitals & Saint
Mary's Health Care System, Grand Rapids,
Michigan; Pediatric Radiology Fellow,
University of Michigan Health System,
Ann Arbor, Michigan

SURESH K. MUKHERJI, MD, FACR
Director of Neuroradiology, Professor and Chief
of Neuroradiology and Head & Neck Radiology;
Professor of Radiology, Otolaryngology Head
Neck Surgery, Radiation Oncology,
Periodontics and Oral Medicine, University of
Michigan Health System, Ann Arbor, Michigan

GOVIND MUKUNDAN, MD
Director of Advanced Imaging, Neuroradiology,
Radiological Associates of Sacramento,
Sacramento, California.

FRANCISCO A. PEREZ, MD, PhD
Department of Radiology, School of Medicine,
University of Washington, Seattle, Washington

PINA C. SANELLI, MD, MPH
Associate Professor, Departments of
Radiology and Public Health, Weill Cornell
Medical College, NewYork-Presbyterian
Hospital, New York, New York

DAVID SEIDENWURM, MD
Neuroradiology, Radiological Associates of
Sacramento, Sacramento, California

MARK S. SHIROISHI, MD
Assistant Professor of Clinical Radiology,
University of Southern California Keck School
of Medicine, Los Angeles, California

PATRICK A. TURSKI, MD, FACR
Professor of Radiology, Neurology and
Neurological Surgery, Division of
Neuroradiology, University of Wisconsin
School of Medicine and Public Health,
Madison, Wisconsin

DAVID M. YOUSEM, MD, MBA
Professor of Radiology, Director of
Neuroradiology, Vice Chairman of Program
Development, Associate Dean of Professional
Development, Russell H. Morgan Department
of Radiology and Radiological Sciences,
Johns Hopkins Medical Institution, Baltimore,
Maryland

Contents

should examine them carefully for opportunities to participate and contribute to ACOs as well as to understand the potential threats. Although there are questions about the viability of the proposed models, neuroradiologists should not assume this is a fad. All specialists should pay close attention to the evolution of ACOs. It seems likely that many of their features will come to pass during the coming decades with substantial impact on the profession.

Certificate of Need (CON) programs represent a patchwork of state regulatory programs across the United States that regulate the availability of selected health care services. Thirty-six states maintain laws designed to ensure access to health care services, maintain or improve quality, and control capital expenditures on health care services and facilities by limiting unnecessary health facility construction and checking the acquisition of major medical equipment. This article discusses the history of CON and explores controversies surrounding the current state of CON regulations.

The paradox of the increased use of imaging without obvious evidence of improved health outcomes has led to calls for payment based on value rather than volume. Measurement of radiologists' performance is a key component of the measurement of value. The paradigm shift occurring in radiology and health care as a whole may seem daunting to the radiologist with the clamor for increasing accountability from payers and patients alike. However, it is through powerful tools such as performance measures in radiology and their accompanying incentive-based payment systems that practices can be improved and confidence of patients restored.

This article provides an overview of the national initiatives developed for monitoring and reporting quality performance measures. Included is a review of the Physician Quality Reporting System, the Hospital Outpatient Quality Data Reporting Program, and the Hospital Outpatient Prospective Payment System, with specific emphasis on how these programs affect radiology practice. A practical review of these programs allows radiologists to gain further understanding of the economic and political influences on the daily practice of radiology today. The background and relevant features of each program are presented in this article.

Expensive advanced imaging, such as magnetic resonance (MR) imaging, contributes to the unsustainable growth of health care costs in the United States. Evidence-based imaging decreases costs and improves outcomes by guiding appropriate utilization of imaging. Low back pain is an important case illustration. Despite strong evidence that early advanced imaging with MR imaging for uncomplicated low back pain leads to increased costs without significant clinical benefit, MR imaging utilization for acute low back pain has increased. Barriers to evidence-based imaging can be traced to patient- and physician-related factors. Radiologists have a critical role in addressing some of these barriers.

Radiology Reporting and Communications: A Look Forward 477

Adam E. Flanders and Paras Lakhani

The content and prose method of radiology reporting has remained essentially unchanged for more than 100 years. By leveraging current technologies, the radiology report has the potential to be a multifunctional document providing information in a number of areas including business analytics, quality assurance and safety, regulatory reporting, research and billing. Maturation and adoption of speech recognition, the development of radiology controlled terminologies and standardized reporting templates now allow for the introduction of structured reporting into the clinical setting.

Combating Overutilization: Radiology Benefits Managers Versus Order Entry Decision Support 497

David M. Yousem

Radiology benefits managers (RBMs) and computerized decision support offer different advantages and disadvantages in the efforts to provide appropriate use of radiology resources. RBMs are effective in their hard-stop ability to reject inappropriate studies, incur a significant cost, and interpose an intermediary between patient and physician. Decision support is a more friendly educational product, but has not been implemented for all clinical indications and its efficacy is still being studied.

Teleradiology 511

William G. Bradley Jr

Picture archiving and communication systems (PACS) and the Internet have changed how clinicians interact with their clinical colleagues, both during the day and at night. Teleradiology may improve the quality of life for radiologists but it also improves the quality of the interpretations for the patients. Given the opportunity this provides to connect subspecialist clinicians with subspecialist radiologists, daytime and nighttime teleradiology is likely to increase. Although teleradiology may worsen the commoditization that started with PACS, patient care will likely be improved, and that should always be the highest priority.

Conflict of Interest in Neuroradiology 519

Patrick A. Turski

A conflict of interest occurs when an outside interest influences professional decisions regarding patient care, education, or research. It is important to recognize conflicts of interest and to report significant financial interests to the appropriate institutional official. When a significant financial interest conflicts with human subjects research, the investigator is typically prohibited from participating in the research. If the conflict does not affect human subjects research, in some instances a conflict of interest management plan can be developed that allows continued participation in the research.

Paul E. Kim and Mark S. Shiroishi

One of the major pitfalls faced by physicians is a basic lack of understanding of the legal aspects of medical malpractice. It is the authors' hope that the brief review of the history of malpractice law provided here affords the radiologist insights that could prove helpful in understanding how one must conduct oneself in a radiology practice. There are several noteworthy points to consider. Vigilance and minimizing errors is always most desirable, but error-free neuroradiology is unattainable. Best medical judgment, although not error free, is at least defensible as noted in the case law discussed here.

Foreword

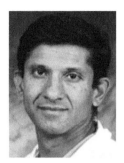

Suresh K. Mukherji, MD, FACR
Consulting Editor

One of the true joys of academics for me has been the opportunity to become colleagues and friends with individuals whom you have admired throughout your career. Dave Yousem was someone who I have respected for many years and who has been a role model for me throughout my career. He is one of those remarkable individuals who excels at everything he does! Dave was one of the first leaders in applying advanced imaging techniques in head and neck cancer. He then went to Hopkins and leads one of the premier neuroradiology divisions in the country and also became one of the youngest presidents of the American Society of Neuroradiology. The "Requisites" is still one of the most popular books in Neuroradiology and one that I reviewed during my preparation for the Neuroradiology Certificate of Added Qualification exam. Dave obtained his Masters of Business Administration and is now focusing his efforts on the socioeconomic aspects of neuroradiology.

This issue of *Neuroimaging Clinics* is a little different from our standard content. However, I felt it was necessary to have such an issue dedicated to neuroradiology given our current political climate and the economic impact neuroradiology has on clinical practice. It is hard to attend a national meeting without having a discussion about the topics discussed in this issue. I was thrilled when Dave agreed to edit this important issue. His passion and enthusiasm for neuroradiology are evident and I am very grateful to him for his extraordinary contribution in creating such an excellent issue.

Suresh K. Mukherji, MD, FACR
Department of Radiology
University of Michigan Health System
1500 East Medical Center
Ann Arbor, MI 48109-0030, USA

E-mail address:
mukherji@med.umich.edu

Neuroimag Clin N Am 22 (2012) xi
doi:10.1016/j.nic.2012.05.017
1052-5149/12/$ – see front matter © 2012 Elsevier Inc. All rights reserved.

Neurolmage: Clinical 00 (2012) 00–00

doi:10.1016/j.nicl.2012.05.012

1053-8119/$ – see front matter © 2012 Elsevier Inc. All rights reserved.

Preface
Socioeconomics of Neuroimaging

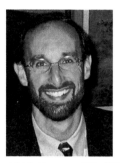

David M. Yousem, MD, MBA
Guest Editor

I am very grateful to Suresh Mukherji for giving me the opportunity to devote an edition of the *Neuroimaging Clinics* to socioeconomics issues. As my career has evolved, the political and financial ramifications of the practice of neuroradiology have become a fascination of mine. The massive economic swings of the last decade in our country have led to tremendous upheaval with respect to the practice of medicine and, in a technology-intensive field such as ours, this has led to pressure to be efficient and well-placed in the market. In academia we are no longer impervious to the shifts in reimbursements and regulations that have led to the instability in the private practice of neuroradiology. On the contrary, we are dealing with performance measures, cost cuts, accountability controls, *in addition* to the issues of graduate medical education, maintenance of certification, fellowship training guidelines, NIH funding cuts, and salary caps. We feel the pain. Trust me. Hopefully this edition of the *Clinics* will provide some tips for navigating through the treacherous paths facing neuroradiologists.

It is always a challenge to assemble a "cast of characters" for a multi-authored contribution to the literature. In this issue you will find many different voices, from a very personal tale by Bill Bradley of his journey through teleradiology to the consultant's voice of Jonathan Berlin and Frank Lexa to the technical side of certificates of need

from Rekha Meesa and Suresh Mukherji. I will say that you should sense from each author, as I did, a sincere enthusiasm in dealing with the topics. These are noted brain, spine, head and neck, MR, CTA, perfusion, embolotherapy experts in neuroradiology who also are passionate about the business and administrative side of the profession. In the past, if you were more operations-oriented in academia, you were discredited by the researchers who considered work even in the social sciences to be fuzzy-wuzzy. Then some great *genius* coined the phrase, "No margin, no mission!" How true. It is only through having a profitable medical system or health care program that our practices, universities, health systems, states, and countries can afford to support the research and development that is required to push our field forward in science. It truly takes a whole village to make a successful health care enterprise. Fortunately, the authors I have included have been innovators in research, clinical care, leadership, education, and business. So you get the whole sh'bang all in one volume!

Hopefully the reader will follow the line of thought in the construction of this volume from practice management to regulation to efficiency to oversight from one article to the next. I have no doubt that you will find invaluable tidbits that will help you in your practice in a different fashion than just a differential diagnosis of a hyperdense

Neuroimag Clin N Am 22 (2012) xiii–xiv
doi:10.1016/j.nic.2012.05.014
1052-5149/12/$ – see front matter

neuroimaging.theclinics.com

posterior fossa mass on NCCT. Understanding the business of neuroradiology will serve you well.

Thank you to the authors (especially for putting up with my incessant reminders!), to the editorial staff, to the support people behind all of our respective careers, to my wife Kelly, to my family, and to the field of neuroradiology, which I love so much.

P.S. (Yes, Kelly I love you even more than the field of neuroradiology.)

David M. Yousem, MD, MBA
Russell H. Morgan Department of
Radiology and Radiological Sciences
The Johns Hopkins Medical Institution
600 N. Wolfe Street, Phipps B100F
Baltimore, MD 21287, USA

E-mail address:
dyousem1@jhu.edu

Strategic Planning for Neuroradiologists

Jonathan W. Berlin, MD, MBA[a],*, Frank J. Lexa, MD, MBA[b,c,d]

KEYWORDS

- Strategic planning • Reimbursement • SWOT • Balanced Scorecard • Radiology economics
- Health care reform

KEY POINTS

- Strategic planning requires an assessment of the current position of a neuroradiology division and a vision of where the neuroradiology would like to be in the near future.
- Two commonly used strategic frameworks are the strengths, weaknesses, opportunities, and threats (SWOT) framework and the balanced scorecard framework, which examines an organization from four perspectives: customer, learning and growth, internal business process, and financial.
- Implementing a strategic plan requires delegation, deadlines, and accountability among those in the organization tasked with implementation.

INTRODUCTION

For many years radiology enjoyed a period of tremendous growth. This advancement was largely due to the advent of new technology, which greatly expanded the diagnostic capabilities of imaging. In neuroradiology, pneumoencephalography became obsolete, and the new cross-sectional modalities of CT and MRI vastly increased the diagnostic armamentarium neuroradiologists use to diagnose central nervous system disorders. New nonimaging medical and surgical technologies also increased patient life expectancies, contributing to higher imaging volume in radiology in general, and in neuroradiology particularly. Between 1999 and 2004, imaging was the fastest growing physician service, and CT and MRI of the central nervous system grew proportionately with other imaging services.[1]

Although the rapid rate of imaging growth dramatically expanded the role of neuroradiology in clinical practice, the expensive nature of neuroimaging was problematic from an economic and strategic planning viewpoint. Technologically sophisticated medical and imaging technologies are cost-intensive, and recently it has become evident that health care expenditures in the United States have increased to the point of potentially being unsustainable. United States health care spending was nearly $2.6 trillion in 2010, over 10 times the amount spent in 1980.[2] To maintain United States competitiveness, increasing attention has been devoted to curbing the growth rate of health care expenditures, with a particular focus on imaging. These economic constraints make effective strategic planning for neuroradiologists essential.

STRATEGIC PLANNING FOR NEURORADIOLOGY

Strategic planning for any organization can be loosely defined as envisioning a future for an organization and working backward to determine a plan of action designed to reach the desired goal.[3] To do so requires several steps that can

[a] Department of Radiology, NorthShore University HealthSystem, 2650 Ridge Avenue, Evanston, IL 60201, USA; [b] Drexel University College of Medicine, 2900 West Queen Lane, Philadelphia, PA 19129, USA; [c] Global Consulting Practicum, The Wharton School, University of Pennsylvania, Vance Hall, 3733 Spruce Street, Philadelphia, PA 19104, USA; [d] Instituto de Empresa, C/ Maria de Molina, 11 28006, Madrid, Spain
* Corresponding author.
E-mail address: jonathanberlin@yahoo.com

Neuroimag Clin N Am 22 (2012) 403–409
doi:10.1016/j.nic.2012.04.007
1052-5149/12/$ – see front matter © 2012 Elsevier Inc. All rights reserved.

be conceptualized as vision, assessment, plan of action, and execution of the plan to achieve the desired goals. Although this methodology intuitively seems straightforward, the strategic planning process is, in fact, difficult. One of the primary reasons is that a desired future cannot be envisioned or achieved in a vacuum; organizations must take stock of the external forces continually influencing them, and at the same time accurately assess their own positive and negative attributes and their willingness and ability to respond to environmental change. Strategic planning also requires prediction and assessment of trends. In radiology in general, and in neuroradiology in particular, this is highly challenging. Commoditization, teleradiology, declining reimbursement, utilization management, political shifts, and technological uncertainty all make the construction of long-standing predictions in neuroradiology problematic (**Box 1**). Not surprisingly, the rapidly evolving health care environment only reinforces the need for neuroradiology leadership organizations to have a cohesive and ongoing strategic planning framework in place.

VISION AND MISSION STATEMENT

A neuroradiology division cannot develop a strategic plan without a vision and mission statement. The vision can be defined as a view of where the neuroradiology division would like to position itself both internally and in the external environment in the present and near future. The mission statement is a written expression of the vision. A good mission statement should be coherent, concise, and timeless, and should elucidate the purpose of the neuroradiology division and its priorities.[4] The mission statement should be familiar to all employees of the neuroradiology division. Superficially, the priorities of a neuroradiology division may seem straightforward: to preserve human life through neuroimaging. However, a deeper examination of the neuroradiology division priorities suggests a more complicated picture, with varying levels of prioritization for the various neuroradiology practice settings. For example, an academic neuroradiology department that relies on a large number of research grants for its financial health may value cutting edge research and peer reviewed publications in addition to, and occasionally more than, a high volume of clinical work. Other less grant-funded academic neuroradiology divisions may place teaching ahead of research, and still other community practice neuroradiology divisions may prioritize clinical output over teaching and research. **Box 2** provides examples of two different mission statements.

Box 1
Selected key uncertainties in neuroradiology

Commoditization: a commodity is defined as a good or service that is only differentiated in the customer's mind by price. If patients see all neuroradiologists as equal in every fashion, they will look toward price as a differentiator.

Teleradiology: teleradiology uses digital picture archiving and communications systems to transport neuroradiology images to an off-site location to be interpreted. When interpretations are moved off-site, other aspects of the role of the neuroradiologist, such as guiding the selection of an appropriate imaging examination, may be overlooked at the primary site.

Declining reimbursement: declining reimbursement can be defined as an overall decrease in payments for radiologic services. Usually this practice is put into place by payors to cut costs.

Utilization management: utilization management in radiology refers to the overseeing of the ordering patterns of radiologic studies by referring physicians through the use of certain criteria that are in some cases proprietary to the utilization manager. Utilization management most often has the effect of decreasing the overall amount of radiology procedures requested.

Political shifts: different political leaders enact policies that influence the overall health care system in a variety of ways, and many policies impact the practice of neuroradiology.

Technological obsolescence: technology is constantly evolving, making some procedures in neuroradiology, such as routine skull examinations, not as clinically useful as other procedures, such as MRI. Shifting technology can influence neuroradiology strategic planning and capital budgeting.

Obviously, no correct and uniform set of goals exists for neuroradiology departments, but priorities of any particular neuroradiology division must be integrated into the mission statement of the neuroradiology department so that strategic decisions align with the overall goals of the neuroradiology section.

A poorly constructed or ambiguous mission statement can contribute to ineffective decisions that do not align with a neuroradiology group's strategic plan. For example, if a neuroradiology division has research as a top priority, taking on a contract to interpret additional off-site neuroimaging studies with the goal of increasing clinical revenue may not be advantageous if it decreases research quality. Conversely, in

---

Box 2
Sample mission statements

Sample Mission Statement One: Our neuroradiology division strives to be a world leader in patient-oriented practice and neuroradiologic technological advancement, including image-based neuroscience and image-guided minimally invasive therapeutics. Our division also strives to provide a state-of-the-art training experience for future neuroradiology leaders.

Comment: With its emphasis on world leadership and teaching, this sample mission statement is probably more typical of an academic neuroradiology division.

Sample Mission Statement Two: Through state-of-the-art technology and clinical excellence, our neuroradiology division strives to provide our patients with the finest neuroradiologic experience in the region.

Comment: With its emphasis on regional dominance and patient experience and clinical excellence, this sample mission statement is probably more typical of a primarily clinical neuroradiology division.

---

a community setting, neuroradiologists might be ill-advised to allocate significant capital expenditures to hire a researcher in lieu of updating their MRI equipment if their mission statement specifies that using state-of-the-art MRI technology is their top priority.

STRATEGIC PLANNING FRAMEWORKS

To plan an appropriate course of action based on a vision requires that organizations take inventory of their own attributes and examine the external environment in which they operate. To help organizations achieve self-awareness, formalized strategic planning frameworks have been developed. Two commonly used strategic planning frameworks are the strengths, weaknesses, opportunities, and threats (SWOT) framework, developed at Harvard University in the late fifties,[5] and the Balanced Scorecard framework, also developed at Harvard in the early nineties.[6] Both strategic planning frameworks are helpful in providing an overall structure to conceptualize strategic planning, yet both have some limitations. The strategic planning frameworks are not mutually exclusive and can be used to complement each other.

THE SWOT FRAMEWORK

Strengths and *weaknesses* are internal attributes that pertain to the neuroradiology division itself, and *opportunities* and *threats* are external environmental attributes that impact the division. For example, an internal strength of a neuroradiology division could be a longstanding ongoing relationship with a leading group of oncologic neurosurgeons in a particular geographic area that leads to a large number of referrals. An internal weakness of a neuroradiology division could be a lack of dedicated outpatient facilities that leads to

a drop in outpatient volume. In contrast, an external threat to a neuroradiology division could be the potential of increased neuroradiology current procedural terminology (CPT) code bundling that will lead to decreased reimbursement on a per case basis. An external opportunity for a neuroradiology division could be nearby geographic areas of high population growth that are currently underserved by neuroradiology.

Assessing internal strengths and weaknesses and external opportunities and threats requires the input of many stakeholders. In neuroradiology, stakeholders are myriad and include payors, patients, radiologists, radiology technologists, vendors, granting agencies, foundations, staff members, business administrators, and referring clinicians. If only one or two stakeholders contribute to identifying an internal strength or weakness, the results can be problematic. For instance, a group of neuroradiologists convening a strategic planning meeting may feel that their customer service is excellent; however, an examination of patient comments from the same neuroradiology practice may cite high wait times or an unfriendly office staff, factors that often correlate with poor customer satisfaction.[7]

As another example, a group of neuroradiologists may feel that a core strength of their organization is 10% annual growth in the volume of brain MRI examinations over the past decade, which they think may ensure their financial success over the next decade. However, at the same time, the billing service fees for this particular neuroradiology practice may have increased and their average days in accounts receivable may have increased, meaning that this neuroradiology division is waiting longer to have their bills paid. Contractual allowances, or the amount discounted from published charges, also may have increased for this practice. In other words, neuroradiologists in this particular practice may feel that their division is doing well financially because their own imaging volume is increasing. However, a broader view of the practice by additional stakeholders, such as business managers or accountants, may show that the financial position of this particular neuroradiology division has in fact become more precarious because of the increase in contractual allowances, the rise in average days in accounts receivable, and the increase in billing service payments.

These examples of perspective difference underscore the need to have a large number of neuroradiology stakeholders participate in identifying organization strengths and weaknesses.

Another limitation of the SWOT framework is that the classification of strengths and weaknesses is somewhat arbitrary.[8] As an example, a neuroradiology division with radiologists who exclusively practice neuroradiology might be considered a strength in a radiology practice large enough to provide the full spectrum of radiologic services in all radiology subspecialties. However, if 24-hour in-house attending radiology service is suddenly required, a radiology department with a neuroradiology division practicing neuroradiology exclusively may experience difficulties with staffing call coverage, because their neuroradiologists might be unable to provide the wide range of non-neuroradiology services needed on an emergent basis. In the scenario in which 24/7 attending radiology coverage is needed in-house, a general radiologist may allow easier scheduling by being able to interpret all types of radiologic studies performed after hours. Another example illustrating the difficulty of classifying an attribute as a strength versus weakness would be a neuroradiology division with a large number of dedicated researchers examining a particular MRI sequence. This group of researchers could be considered a strength in that greater expertise is developed in a particular MRI sequence, but could also be seen as a weakness if this division might be less receptive to MRI protocol changes that may be needed. Information gleaned from external neuroradiology divisions may prove valuable when working within the SWOT framework. For example, a neuroradiology division might initially perceive a particular new 3T MRI unit as a huge opportunity for expanding their clinical volume, but a site visit to another neuroradiology division using that particular 3T unit may reveal suboptimal image quality, which could present a significant obstacle to expanding clinical volume. Occasionally, external consultants may also be engaged to assess the potential for a new strategic opportunity or the validity of a perceived external threat for a neuroradiology division, such as a new marketing or branding campaign, or a new local or national competitor.

However, the SWOT framework may not take into account a company's entire strategic snapshot. For example, the SWOT framework can leave out the financial and operational components of an organization if it is not performed thoroughly. Therefore, the SWOT framework exclusively may not be sufficient to construct a contemporary inventory of a neuroradiology division's status for strategic planning. SWOT, however, is useful in that it provides a skeleton of important department attributes from which to work. Box 3 provides a summary list of important positive and negative attributes of the SWOT framework.

BALANCED SCORECARD

Other strategic planning frameworks, such as the Balanced Scorecard, can complement the SWOT framework (see Box 3). The Balanced

---

Box 3
Selected key summary points for SWOT and balanced scorecard frameworks

Key Positive and Negative Attributes of the SWOT Framework

Positive attributes

- Easy to understand
- Provides a basic framework for thinking about strategic planning
- Straightforward analysis

Negative attributes

- Classification of strengths and weaknesses can be arbitrary
- May not provide a complete picture of a neuroradiology division
- Completion requires input of a variety of stakeholders

Key Strengths and Weaknesses of the Balanced Scorecard Framework

Strengths

- Takes into account financial and nonfinancial factors
- Takes into account operations and employee growth and engagement

Weaknesses

- Primarily an internal assessment
- May neglect external factors

Scorecard examines a business from four distinct perspectives: the customer, the internal business process, the financial, and the learning and growth perspectives.[9]

The customer perspective examines the enterprise from the perspective of a customer. In the case of neuroradiology, this perspective would focus on factors known to correlate with patient and referring clinician satisfaction, such as wait times for the performance and results of an imaging study.[10] The financial perspective examines the neuroradiology division from the perspective of an auditor. This analysis would require an examination of the type of examinations performed, the reimbursement received for each examination, the trends in revenue receipt and payor policies for neuroradiology procedures, and a cost analysis of the neuroradiology section.

The business process perspective examines the neuroradiology section from the perspective of operations, addressing the question of what business systems enhance or slow down the process between the time a referring physician orders a neuroradiology examination and the time that same referring physician has the results of the examination they ordered in their office. Potential operational bottlenecks, or rate-limiting steps, in a neuroradiology section may include a long interval between the time a CT or MRI examination is completed and when it is sent to a picture archiving and communication system (PACS system) in a verified status to be interpreted. Occasionally, bottlenecks can also occur if there is a long wait to load a comparison study on PACS.

The perspective of learning and growth examines corporate culture and employee training to assess the ease with which an organization can change and maneuver to meet its goals. Viewing a neuroradiology collective from a learning and growth perspective might entail examining the speed at which diffusion imaging was introduced into a particular neuroradiology division. To do this would require an examination of the availability and opportunity for technologists and radiology attending physicians to participate in continuing medical education devoted to diffusion imaging, and would assess whether the employees and partners of the neuroradiology division believed that they had the tools to perform their jobs in a superb manner. A neuroradiology section reluctant to modify its protocols or hesitant to offer technologist training in diffusion imaging might score low from a learning and growth perspective. In addition to facilitating innovation, attention to the learning and growth perspective should optimize employee engagement or involvement, thus facilitating the translation of vision into action.

Box 3 presents a brief summary of the strengths and weaknesses of the Balanced Scorecard framework.

COMMON THEMES OF STRATEGIC PLANNING FRAMEWORKS

Strategic planning frameworks such as SWOT and Balanced Scorecard are valuable in that they provide a structure for conceptualizing the place of a neuroradiology section in the environment. They allow the stakeholders to obtain an adequate foothold on how the department or division is functioning at a given time in relation to its environment. This knowledge, in conjunction with a solid vision, is essential to strategic planning. However, successful strategic planning also requires translating an organization's vision and self-awareness into action.

TRANSLATING THE STRATEGIC VISION INTO ACTION

In many cases, the creation of a mission statement and the drafting of a proposed course of action is the easy part of strategic planning. Too often, once created, the proposed plan of action is only dreamed about rather than executed (**Fig. 1**). Putting the plan into action is often difficult, but is an essential step in strategic planning.

Important steps in ensuring execution of the strategic plan are communication, delegation, deadlines, accountability, and open communication among parties involved in the strategic plan (see **Box 4**).[11] First and foremost, the strategic

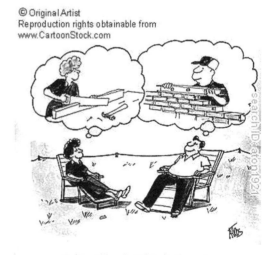

© Original Artist
Reproduction rights obtainable from
www.CartoonStock.com

Jack and Ina build their dream house

Fig. 1. The tendency to dream, rather than execute, a plan of action. (*From* CartoonStock. Available at: www.cartoonstock.com; used with permission.)

plan and proposed course of action should be communicated to everyone involved in its execution. For a neuroradiology division, this will likely include neuroradiologists and technologists, administrators, secretaries, and office staff. All appropriate neuroradiology division employees should be familiar with not only the proposed course of action but also the reason for the new or modified course.

Delegation of responsibilities is also essential to the implementation of a strategic plan. For example, if a neuroradiology strategic plan calls for decreasing outpatient wait times by 10%, a specific neuroradiology employee or team, possibly a manager or management team, should be tasked with this goal. That person or team's job should be to determine an appropriate course of action needed to fulfill the goal, and that person or team's responsibility should be to ensure that the goal is performed. To facilitate implementation of the goal, the person or team tasked with this purpose must have the tools to track the progress. People charged with implementing the strategic plan also need to have the support of the senior neuroradiology leadership to motivate employees needed to implement the plan. For example, deceasing neuroradiology outpatient wait times would be impossible without a mechanism in place to track these wait times, and decreasing wait times may be very difficult without the ability to incentivize employees to do so. To incentivize employees, a neuroradiology division might promise a financial bonus or additional time off if wait times decrease in the desired manner. Internal award or recognition mechanisms, such as

personal congratulations for a job well done, can also be effective in some cases to motivate employees to executive the strategic plan.

Deadlines are also important when executing a strategic plan. Those tasked with implementing a step in the plan should know how long they have to institute this implementation. For example, a neuroradiology division seeking to improve the friendliness of its office staff might set the goal of improving patient satisfaction scores in the area of office friendliness within 6 months from the time the goal is communicated to the person or people tasked with its implementation. Frequent monitoring of progress in the strategic plan execution is also important, as is review by, and appropriate feedback from, the senior management team.[12]

Strategic plan implementation also means holding those tasked with fulfilling certain goals responsible if those goals are not met in the appropriate time frame.[13] Holding people accountable for fulfilling goals may mean that a promotion or a bonus does not occur if the goal was not met. However, open communication between those delegated with performing a goal and senior management to assess potentially valid reasons for the lack of goal fulfillment also should be in place. For example, if adequate tracking mechanisms were not established to monitor wait times, concluding that wait times were not decreased because of poor employee performance may be inappropriate.

Strategic Planning for an Uncertain Future

The changing health care system is accompanied by uncertainties for neuroradiology divisions. The evolving delivery of health care may necessitate a gradual culture change among neuroradiologists (Box 1). Traditionally, physician autonomy has been paramount in medical practice. In neuroradiology, this autonomy might translate into neuroradiologists requesting a particular MRI sequence for an examination to evaluate for multiple sclerosis that is different from their colleagues. It might also translate into neuroradiologists who do not use voice recognition or do not self-edit their radiology reports when their colleagues do. In a future system in which standardization, coordination, teamwork, and efficiency are valued, all physicians, including neuroradiologists, may need to change their methods of practice. It will be incumbent on neuroradiology leaders to facilitate this culture change so that an effective strategic plan for their organization can be realized.[14]

CONCLUDING THOUGHTS

The translation of an effective strategic plan for neuroradiology will require knowledge of the internal and external environment and the vantage points provided by the balanced scorecard. It will also require vision and a thoroughly internalized and communicated mission statement to guide decision making. Effective neuroradiology leadership will be essential in executing a well-thought-out strategic plan and will give those tasked with strategic plan execution the tools and incentives to implement the plan. It is also important to realize that strategic planning is ongoing, and neuroradiology departments and divisions will need to remain flexible to cope with the rapidly changing environment. To that end, neuroradiologists should educate themselves on the constantly evolving economic and societal trends influencing health care delivery. This awareness will facilitate the process of effective strategic planning, leadership, and an appropriate action plan based on a well-thought-out ongoing strategic planning process.

TAKE HOME POINTS

1. Neuroradiology departments need a vision and mission statement. The vision is a conceptualization of where the neuroradiology division would like to be in the near future, and the mission statement is a written encapsulation of the vision.
2. After creating the vision and drafting the mission statement, neuroradiology groups should take an inventory of their positive and negative attributes.
3. SWOT and Balanced Scorecard are strategic planning frameworks that can be used by neuroradiology departments to assess their position in the environment. They are not mutually exclusive, and groups should feel free to also use other frameworks.
4. Multiple stakeholders are needed to generate a complete list of a neuroradiology division's positive and negative attributes.
5. SWOT stands for strengths, weaknesses, opportunities, and threats. Strengths and weaknesses are internal, and pertain to the neuroradiology department exclusively. Opportunities and threats are external, and pertain to the environment that affects the neuroradiology department.
6. Balanced Scorecard is a strategic framework that views an organization from four distinct vantage points: the customer perspective; the internal business process, or operations, perspective; the financial perspective; and the learning and growth perspective.
7. Effective translation of a strategic plan into action requires dynamic leadership.

8. In the future, the practice of neuroradiology may involve utilization management and increased collaboration with nonradiology colleagues in addition to the interpretation of radiologic examinations.
9. Neuroradiology leaders will likely lead a major shift in the culture of neuroradiology. The new culture may require neuroradiologists to work as part of a multispecialty central nervous system team.
10. Putting a strategic plan into action requires communication, delegation, deadlines, and accountability. It also requires that senior leadership provide the appropriate tools for strategic plan execution.

REFERENCES

1. MedPac Recommendation on Imaging Services. Available at: http://www.medpac.gov/documents/071806_Testimony_imaging.pdf. Accessed November 6, 2011.
2. US Health care costs. Available at: http://www.kaiseredu.org/Issue-Modules/US-Health-Care-Costs/Background-Brief.aspx. Accessed October 27, 2011.
3. Business Directory. Available at: http://www.businessdictionary.com/definition/strategic-planning.html. Accessed June 5, 2012.
4. Vogt J. Demystifying the mission statement. Nonprof World 1994;12(1):29–32.
5. Panagiotou G. Bringing SWOT into focus. Bus Strat Rev 2003;14(2):8–10.
6. Kaplan RS, Norton DP. Using the balanced scorecard as a strategic management system. Harv Bus Rev 2007;150–61.
7. White B. Measuring patient satisfaction: how to do it and why bother. Fam Pract Manag 1999;6:40–4.
8. Grant MR. Contemporary strategy analysis—concepts, techniques, applications. 4th edition. Malden, MA: Blackwell Publishing; 2002.
9. Grigoroudis E, Orfanoudaki E, Zopounidis C. Strategic performance measurement in a healthcare organisation; a multiple criteria approach based on balanced scorecard. Omega 2011;40:104–19.
10. Basu PA, Ruiz-Wibbelsmann JA, Spielman SB, et al. Creating a patient-centered imaging service: determining what patients want. AJR Am J Roentgenol 2011;196:605–10.
11. Raffoni M. Three keys to effective execution. Harv Manag Update 2008;13(6):3–4.
12. Gee M. Three simple steps to activate your strategic plan. Nonprof World 2008;26(5):14.
13. Neilson G, Martin K, Powers E. The secrets to successful strategy execution. Harv Bus Rev 2008;86:61–70.
14. Lee TH. Turning doctors into leaders. Harv Bus Rev 2010;88:50–8.

Turf Issues in Radiology and Its Subspecialties

Jacqueline Bello, MD

KEYWORDS

- Turf issues • Radiology • Quality of care • Patient safety • Radiology training • Self referral
- Imaging utilization

KEY POINTS

- Turf issues affect policy, practice, and patients.
- Contributing/connected factors include control of patients, self-referral, and overuse.
- Turf issues impact quality of care and patient safety.
- Proposed strategies for radiology confronting turf issues center on accreditation of facilities; standardization of training; formulation of a structured, clinically rich subspecialty curriculum; multispecialty collaboration in the development of practice guidelines; expansion of radiology research; and endorsement of legislation *against* self-referral and *for* certificate of need.
- Radiology's continued relevance depends on a patient-centered focus and maintaining clinical excellence, including specialty and subspecialty expertise.

> *"Nothing in life is to be feared, it is only to be understood."*
>
> *–Marie Curie*

INTRODUCTION

Beyond mere politics, turf issues in medicine affect policy, practice, and, most importantly, patients. This article explores the issue of turf from several perspectives. The discourse begins by defining the issue and scope of the problem, followed by a brief history of turf delineation. Consideration of contributing and connected factors further frame this discussion, which then takes into account some of the consequences of turf battles and their impact on related topics. Finally, concentration focuses on proposed strategies to successfully confront the questions, if not overcome the problems raised by these issues. To better inform the deliberation and strengthen the credibility of any conclusions, the evidence and controversies must be regarded from beyond merely the radiology perspective.

TURF DELINEATION AND SCOPE OF THE PROBLEM

A 2002 Web site survey of radiologists identified turf battles as the second largest problem threatening the field, after manpower shortage (http://www. auntminnie.com).[1] Radiologists' claim to turf is predicated on the fact that they are the only physicians whose training includes 4 to 6 years of education dedicated to imaging science, technology, and safety; imaging protocols; image interpretation with clinical correlation; and performance of image-guided procedures. Conversant in the language of all imaging modalities, radiologists are well positioned to designate the appropriate examination for the clinical question, and tailor the protocol for the study.

Debates over turf issues may extend beyond the chair and faculty of a competing specialty to include hospital and medical school administrations, boards of trustees, insurance carriers, and legislators. By expansion, the political debate shifts from the professional arena to include stakeholders well beyond it.

Department of Radiology, Montefiore Medical Center, 111 East 210th Street, Bronx, NY 10467-2490, USA
E-mail address: JBELLO@montefiore.org

Neuroimag Clin N Am 22 (2012) 411–419
doi:10.1016/j.nic.2012.04.006
1052-5149/12/$ – see front matter © 2012 Elsevier Inc. All rights reserved.

HISTORICAL PERSPECTIVE

A brief review of the history of turf delineation is important from the standpoint of understanding the issue at hand, in addition to gaining insight into how to deal with it.[2] Coronary angiography was developed by radiology physicians Judkins and Amplatz in the sixties, and was performed by radiologists through the seventies, but almost none is performed by radiologists today.[3,4] Although coronary angiography represents the first "lost art" suffered by radiology,[5] it is noteworthy that the initial Resource-Based Relative Value Scale (RBRVS) instituted for Medicare in 1992 allowed payment for interpretations by cardiology *and* radiology when both were involved in providing the service. At that time, the Current Procedural Terminology (CPT) description of the service was vague enough that two distinct interpretations could be performed and billed. Medicare then developed component coding that separated the "doing" of the procedure from "supervising and interpreting" the procedure, allowing for only a single interpretation of the angiogram. Cardiologists could bill one or both parts, but if cardiology did both, this prevented the radiologist from submitting a billable interpretation. In essence, radiology's interpretation, and therefore the radiologist, became unnecessary to the process. Furthermore, a current focus of the Centers for Medicare and Medicaid Services (CMS) is to reduce component coding (or in some cases abolish it altogether) and "bundle" the procedural and interpretative portions of certain examinations. Therefore, when two separate specialties perform the separate components, the history of lost coronary angiography could easily be repeated.

Today, turf battles exist throughout the scope of radiology's practice, in ultrasound (including echocardiography, obstetrics, prostate, vascular, and emergency department studies); skeletal and chest radiography; bone densitometry and cardiac nuclear studies; urinary, musculoskeletal, and vascular interventions; and neurointerventions. In some areas of the country, diagnostic neuroradiology's high relative value unit procedures are also being claimed by neurologists, neurosurgeons, and orthopedic surgeons. Neuroimaging fellowships developed by neurologists and accredited through non–Accreditation Council for Graduate Medical Education (ACGME) societies have been established in many locales.

These battles also exist outside the scope of radiology practice, such as between orthopedic spine surgeons and neurosurgeons over spine surgery; gastroenterologists and colorectal surgeons over colonoscopy; and dermatology and surgeons over minor plastic procedures.

The fact that physicians work within the economic confines of a "zero sum game" necessarily creates competition and friction among specialties. Historically, this fact derives from the Balanced Budget Act of 1997, and 15 years later continues to fuel turf battles as one of the major contributing factors.[6]

CONTRIBUTING AND CONNECTED FACTORS

Control of patients is not the purview of radiologists. In addition, most radiologists lack clinical training and expertise in the medical subspecialties encroaching on their turf. A clear disconnect often exists between the radiologist and the patient, and the radiology report is at best a surrogate for interaction with clinical colleagues. These factors undermine the radiologist's position in deliberations over turf management (**Box 1**). They also help explain why the radiologist is often overlooked, an invisible link in the chain that begins with a symptom, leads to diagnosis of disease, and continues through its treatment, and control, if not cure, in follow-up care.

Self-referral promotes turf battles and is also a major contributor to over use. In a 2003 report to Congress, the Medicare Payment Advisory Commission (MedPAC) reviewed growth in Medicare services from 1999 to 2002 in four categories of service: evaluation and management, medical tests, procedures, and imaging. Imaging was at the forefront of growth, advancing at a rate more than twice that for procedures![7] Research by Hillman and colleagues[8,9] showed that self-referred imaging by nonradiologist physicians increased 1.7 to 7.7 times the amount of imaging referred to radiologists by nonradiologist physicians for the same clinical conditions. Similar research was reported by the U.S. General Accounting Office (GAO), clearly unbiased, and certainly not reported from a radiologist's perspective. The GAO compared imaging use rates according to modality for nonradiologist physicians with in-office imaging equipment versus rates for nonradiologist

---

Box 1
Factors contributing to radiology turf issues

- Clinical "control" of patients
- Self-referral by nonradiology physicians
- Auto-referral by radiologists
- Training requirements of nonradiology specialty boards

physicians who referred the imaging to radiologists. For 19.4 million office visits generating 3.5 million imaging studies, they found the rates to be 1.95% to 5.13% higher in the self-referred group.[10] In response to these data, nonradiologist physicians offered rationales for self-referred imaging. Temple[11] argued that the nonradiologist imager can better integrate the clinical data, and further suggested that self-referred outpatient imaging may be less expensive than referral to a hospital radiology department. Burris and Mroczek[11] noted that if requesting physicians had to refer studies rather than perform them, they may not take the time and effort to do so. Grajower[11] stated that patients expect/insist that their own physician perform the imaging. Inconvenience to patients having to take additional time off work and inconvenience to physicians having to wait for results to begin treatment have also been cited in arguments rationalizing self-referral.[11,12]

Maintaining objectivity, it is only fair to acknowledge that the self-referral finger also has been pointed at radiologists.[12] The term *auto-referral* has been used to describe this practice, which was studied in a systematic review of 545 consecutive CT scans of the abdomen and in tracking recommendations made for additional imaging. Although these recommendations were made in 19% of cases, they were performed in only 30% of these, or 6% of the entire group. This figure for auto-referral is considerably less than those reported for self-referral by nonradiologists performing imaging on their own equipment.[13] Auto-referral differs from self-referral in the context of viewing the radiologist as a consultant. In fact, initial assessments by clinical consultants often are not definitive, and further workup, including additional testing, is recommended. Similarly, called on to consult through imaging, a radiologist is equally justified in recommending further studies to facilitate diagnosis.[14]

Additional contributing factors to the battle for turf stem from the fact that certain nonradiology subspecialty board examinations require training in various diagnostic and interventional aspects of radiology. This exposure opens the door to encroachment at an early stage of practice, during training. Similarly, allied research, which is common in radiology, offers the opportunity for clinical colleagues to acquaint themselves with advanced imaging techniques on a level that surpasses mere clinical utility/interest. In some cases, primary research within a clinical subspecialty may be ahead of the trajectory that radiology is taking toward the same goal. Finally, as outcomes in health care become increasingly important, clinicians not only adopt imaging metrics but are also seeking to help define them.

CONSEQUENCES AND IMPACT OF TURF BATTLES

Deeply intertwined in the discussion of turf, the issues of self-referral and overuse raise concern over quality of care and, ultimately, patient safety (Box 2). The accuracy of self-referred interpretations has been questioned, both within and outside the radiology literature.[15] One study compared the readings of 60 chest radiographs with proven diagnoses by three separate panels: the first comprising radiologists with board certification, the second having radiology residents, and the third having nonradiologist physicians. Statistically significant difference among the panels was shown by receiver operating characteristic curve analysis, with the nonradiologist physicians performing least well. Notably, the radiology residents on the second panel had a mean length of training of 2.4 years.[16] A separate study from an academic medical center used four physician panels; the first included faculty radiologists, the second had radiology residents, the third had emergency medicine faculty, and the fourth had emergency medicine residents. They interpreted a film set of 120 radiographs of the chest, abdomen and skeletal system, approximately half of which had clinically significant findings. The study reported an overall accuracy of 80% for radiology faculty, 71% for radiology residents, 59% for emergency medicine faculty, and 57% for emergency medicine residents.[17] Because plain films are considered to be less complex than CT, MRI, or sonography, the differences in each of these studies probably would have been greater if they included the more complex examinations. A review of 555 studies compared head CT interpretations by emergency department physicians to interpretations by radiologists. Misinterpretation by emergency department physicians occurred in 24% of cases, and included missed abnormalities, such as infarcts, masses, cerebral edema, parenchymal hemorrhages, contusions, and subarachnoid hemorrhages.[18] The publication of the Institute of Medicine's report *To Err is Human: Building a Safer Health System*[19] focuses attention on the reduction

---

Box 2
Impact of radiology turf issues

- Overuse of imaging (by nonradiologist imagers)

- Image quality and accuracy of image interpretation (by nonradiologist imagers)

- Health care cost increase (from repeat examinations)

of medical errors and improvement of patient safety. The evidence showing that more accurate interpretations of imaging studies are given by radiologists than nonradiologist physicians should be factored into the debate over who should perform the interpretation. This finding is increasingly important as health care reform efforts attempt to replace volume with value with a focus on quality and safety measures.

Poor quality of services accounts for approximately 30% of health care costs in the United States, to the tune of approximately $390 billion per year.[20] Inadequate image quality leads to repeat examinations, which inevitably results in increased imaging costs. Repeat examinations also inconvenience patients, and may expose them to additional radiation. A quality audit of in-office radiology services conducted by Pennsylvania Blue Shield across various specialties showed that radiology and orthopedic providers had relatively low rates of unacceptable image quality, at 12% to 13% compared with 41% to 82% for internal medicine, pulmonary medicine, podiatry, and chiropractic providers.[21] Image quality is just one aspect of quality care. Blue Cross Blue Shield of Massachusetts addressed additional factors through a site inspection study of more than a thousand outpatient imaging facilities. The additional components of quality considered by the study were staff training and qualifications, equipment specifications and performance, quality control procedures, records management and storage, and safety procedures. Among the sites, 20% failed the inspection, with deficiencies that were deemed to be correctable. An additional 11% of the sites failed inspection because of serious fundamental issues, and were suspended from reimbursement. Inspection pass rates were highest for radiologists, cardiologists, and mobile units at 95%, and lowest for internists, podiatrists, and chiropractors at less than 62%.[22,23] Recent trends in manufacturing less expensive equipment may result in lower quality. Convenience and financial incentive help sell equipment that is easily available to nonradiologist physicians, such as extremity-only MRI units and handheld ultrasound units. The portability of this equipment easily places it outside of radiology, and further blurs margins of turf.

To ensure the quality and safety of equipment, the American College of Radiology (ACR) has established accreditation programs in 10 different imaging modalities. Since 1987, the ACR has accredited more than 20,000 facilities, including more than 10,000 practices. In 2008, under the Medicare Improvements for Patients and Providers Act (MIPPA), CMS mandated accreditation of certain imaging modalities to qualify for reimbursement.[24] This CMS mandate opened the door for turf battles to extend into the accreditation arena. In 2002, the American College of Cardiology joined with other specialties, including neurology, neurosurgery, and orthopedic surgery, to form the Intersocietal Commission for the Accreditation of Magnetic Resonance Laboratories (ICAMRL) for the accreditation of facilities.[1]

Turf battles raise another important question, that of training in diagnostic imaging and how much is enough?[25] As a result of imaging being performed outside of radiology, many nonradiology medical specialty societies have produced training standards for diagnostic imaging. From the perspective of radiology, tremendous variation exists among these standards, which are generally the product of a consensus panel, and range from being lenient to strict.[26] The issue has relevance beyond turf, as MedPAC and commercial payers begin to look to these standards for reimbursement of physicians performing and reporting imaging studies.[27] In addition, the ACR is building a program for physicians to be trained and designated as providers of medical imaging for reimbursement purposes.[28]

Several studies have documented that board certified radiologists and radiology residents in training outperform nonradiologist physicians in interpreting standardized image sets. Moreover, within radiology itself, the accuracy of interpretation has been shown to correlate with the level of training of the interpreting radiologist. To this end, Wechsler and colleagues[29] compared second- and third-year radiology resident overnight reads and cross-sectional imaging fellow reads versus final attending interpretations of emergency body CT scans. Discrepancy in readings was classified as major or minor. For the resident cases, the major discrepancy rate was 2.8% and the minor discrepancy rate was 10.6%, and for the fellows, these rates were 0.7% and 5.3%, respectively. Their obvious conclusion was that in film interpretation, radiologists in their fifth year of training by far exceeded those with only 2 or 3 years of training in performance. A study in ultrasound training tracked the sequential progress made by 10 first-year residents at the benchmarks of having performed their first 50, 100, 150, and 200 cases. The test consisted of performing and interpreting 10 cases, and a passing grade for each case required demonstration of 80% of required landmarks and making no clinically significant interpretation errors. After 200 cases, the mean number of clinically significant errors per case was 0.5 (range, 0.2–1.0) and the mean percentage of passed cases was 16% (range, 0%–50%). The clear conclusion was that evaluation of more than 200 cases is needed to achieve competence in the performance and interpretation of ultrasound. Based on these data, the ACR and the American Institute of Ultrasound in Medicine have both established minimum training requirements of at least 500 ultrasound examinations.[30]

This example of cooperative effort in establishing rigorous standards should preserve the dimensions of quality and safety for patients by allowing turf access only to experienced operators. Unfortunately, in 2000, the American Medical Association House of Delegates passed policy H-230.960, placing ultrasound within the scope of practice of *any* "appropriately trained physician," recommending that hospital staff credentialing be based on standards developed by the *physician's* specialty.[26,31] This description leaves the question of appropriate training purposefully vague, and neither protects turf nor the quality of care.

Lastly, in examining how turf battles impact training, studies evaluating the effect of training at higher levels of physician experience are considered. Second readings provided by two subspecialty radiologists reviewing outside CT scans on 143 patients with known cancer were compared with the initial readings provided by general radiologists. In 17% of cases, the subspecialty read differed significantly from the initial read, and included previously undiagnosed lymphadenopathy, pulmonary nodules, hepatic lesions, and extrahepatic masses.[32] In a similar study conducted at four academic cancer centers, subspecialty second readings disagreed with initial reads in 41% of cases. Final diagnoses, established through surgery, biopsy, or 6-month clinical and imaging follow-up, confirmed the second subspecialty read to be correct in 92% of the discrepant cases, the initial read to be correct in 6%, and neither to be correct in 2%.[33] Training and experience matters at all levels of training and practice, and clearly impacts quality.

STRATEGIES TO FACE THE ISSUES

In his 2006 ACR presidential oration, Dr Milton Guiberteau stressed the importance of radiology maintaining its relevance in today's health care system. To raise "doing a job" to the level of a profession, he invoked the concept of a "job with a conscience," citing three primary responsibilities as critical to the concept: duty to patients radiologists serve; duty to society, at whose pleasure radiologists serve; and duty to colleagues with whom radiologists serve, and thereby the profession itself.[34] Strategies to protect the profession must keep the patient's best interest and the

greater good of society central to the discussion (**Box 3**). In many instances, advocacy on behalf of patients may help protect turf. For example, advocating that patients are entitled to have imaging studies and image-guided procedures performed by properly trained physicians is mutually beneficial. Placing emphasis on appropriateness in imaging will benefit patients and society through reducing redundant testing, unwarranted radiation exposure, and avoidable costs. Implemented effectively, this strategy would curtail self-referral and imaging overuse as secondary benefits.

In confronting challenges posed by turf battle, the following specific strategies have been proposed,[35,36] many of which stem from the contributing and connected issues, and the consequences and impact issues that have been presented.

Endorsement of Mandatory Accreditation of Imaging Facilities

In addition to facility standards of equipment performance and maintenance, quality assurance and control, radiation safety, outcomes analyses, film and report quality, and record keeping, this accreditation would include strict training and experience requirements for technologists and medical physicists. Enforcement of standards would disqualify imaging providers not meeting them.

Enforcement of Physician Training Standards for Imaging/Image-Guided Interventions

Radiology resident and fellowship training programs undergo ACGME accreditation. The neuroradiology fellowship accreditation standards were formally recognized by the ACGME in 1991, and subspecialty certification in neuroradiology, with a 10-year renewable certificate of added qualification (CAQ), has been offered since 1995.

Box 3
Survival strategies for radiologists

- Equipment accreditation
- Training standards
- Practice guidelines
- Legislation supporting certificate of need
- Legislation against self-referral
- Expansion of research
- Patient-centered focus
- Imaging privileging and decision support

More than 85 academic institutions sponsor the 200+ fellowship positions in the United States annually.[37] Fellowship training programs in neuroimaging, established by neurologists, have been accredited through a non-ACGME "umbrella group" of neurology professional organizations, the United Council of Neurologic Subspecialities, and this council designated neuroimaging as the sixth subspecialty of neurology in 2006. Concern has been raised over misaligned incentives and risk for self-referral and overuse by neurologist owners of imaging centers.[7,8,38] Moreover, exposure to a large volume of cases that is rich in both variety and acuity of pathology is the lynchpin of neuroimaging training. An analysis of Medicare data showed that radiologists interpret most (98.3%) neuroimaging studies and that the limited exposure that neurologists have to CT and MR examinations could only support 12 fellowship positions based on the ACGME standards of 1500 MRI and 1500 CT examinations per year, per fellow.[37]

To impact the level at which the "bar" is set, radiology organizations must be more involved in collaboration with other specialties to develop rigorous training standards for physicians. The multidisciplinary approach lends objectivity and credibility to the process, giving the end result some "legs" for its application to required elements for reimbursement.

Creation of a Formal Radiology Curriculum

Current training requirements for residents in diagnostic radiology are only broadly defined by the ACGME in the Graduate Medical Education Directory, also known as the green book.[39] Subspecialty expertise is becoming increasingly important in turf protection from clinical subspecialists performing and/or interpreting imaging studies. Redefining the residency to include a core curriculum and an advanced training period has been proposed, and the timing of the American Board of Radiology examination is being "re-set" so the final examination will occur a year after completion of residency, as is the case for most other specialties.[40] Expertise and experience form the foundation of the subspecialty radiologist's strategy in turf struggles with clinical subspecialists. For example, a neuroradiologist may offer a differential diagnosis that includes non-neurologic conditions based on their more general training. Neuroradiologists, by training, are more capable of multimodality correlation than their clinical neuroscience colleagues, and have a richer lexicon of artifacts and normal variants in neuroimaging. In addition, neuroradiologists are more

acutely aware of radiation and MR safety implications when recommending further examinations. Finally, through maintenance of subspecialty certification, neuroradiologists keep pace with advances in imaging technology.[41]

Acquisition of Clinical and Pathology Expertise by Radiologists

As delivery of care necessarily becomes more patient-centered, strong clinical knowledge is increasingly important to radiologists. In addition, more clinical and pathology expertise will be needed by radiologists to gain access to the developing turf of molecular imaging.

Being "one step removed" from the patient only diminishes the relevance of the radiologist. Radiologists need to reconnect with patients and be recognized as not only one of their doctors but also the doctor central to the other doctors credited with the diagnosis and cure. Clinical rounding to demonstrate imaging findings and participate in next-step decision making for inpatients, and holding diagnostic imaging clinics that share results with outpatients, have been proposed as solutions to bring the radiologist back into the picture.[42] (This would give a whole new meaning to the term film credits.)

Multispecialty Practice Guideline Development for Imaging

As with the development of training standards, practice guideline development should include input from other specialties to determine what imaging studies, if any, are appropriate for a given clinical situation. The ACR Appropriateness Criteria provide a firm foundation for the development of clinical decision rules for imaging, which would also be valuable to regulatory agencies.[43] Radiology taking an active role in helping control imaging use is important in convincing policy makers, payers, and health care administrators that radiologists provide the critical difference in expertise required for imaging decisions.

Expansion of Radiology Research

Promoting high-quality imaging research is essential for radiology to maintain a presence and relevance in today's practice of medicine. In the words of Bruce Hillman, MD, head of the ACR Imaging Network, "Especially given the relentless encroachment on imaging by other specialists, it seems incontrovertible... that our continued success as a specialty will principally depend on our research capacity to develop and demonstrate the benefit of further innovations."[44] An effective strategy for defending against turf encroachment is showing leadership and expertise through ground-breaking, high-level research. Emphasis must be placed on multicenter clinical trials to define best practices in radiology and evaluate clinical outcomes for radiologist practices compared with those of nonradiologist physicians.[45] Given the effect that economic constraints place on research, the suggestion has even been made that, for the greater good of radiology, private practice contribution to the funding of research would be reasonable.[46] James Borgstede, MD, past chairman of the ACR Board of Chancellors, has aptly stated, "The specialty performing the research is likely to be the specialty putting the research into practice."[47] Coming in at the ground level of research certainly helps stake a claim on ownership of the turf.

Legislation Against Self-Referral

The all-too-familiar loophole in the Stark laws limiting self-referral, the in-office ancillary services exemption, actually helps promote self-referral, and as a result, turf battles. At the state level, this has been addressed by Maryland, where limiting self-referral according to the Maryland Health Occupations Article 1-301(k)(2) has met with some success. Other states, including Texas and Indiana, are attempting to follow suit.

Precertification of Self-Referred Examinations, Audit Provisions

Statistics cited previously showed that from two to eight times the imaging volume was performed by self-referred physicians compared with radiologists for the same clinical condition.[7] Those same data deem that from 40% to 50% of self-referred examinations are unnecessary. Therefore, requiring that precertification be hinged to reimbursement for self-referred examinations would be a reasonable initiative. Alternative suggestions call for withholding the professional component of reimbursement for these examinations, paying only the technical component, in an effort to decrease any financial incentive behind them.[48,49] Audit provisions would allow payers, including government agencies, access to physician records to review the actual clinical indications for self-referred examinations and compare them with the indications used for precertification. Discovery of discrepancies would incur penalties, an obvious "stick" versus "carrot" approach to dissuade phony indications contrived for precertification purposes.[36]

Endorsement of Imaging Privileging Programs

Some of the accreditation programs include restricting the privileges of nonradiologist imaging providers to perform only certain types of examinations. One program in Connecticut disallowed cardiologists from performing non-cardiac ultrasound, nuclear medicine, and radiography, and limited orthopedic surgeons to performing skeletal radiography, but not MRI. Implementation of this program resulted in a 32% decrease in billing of payers by nonradiologist physicians who either failed site inspections with limitations on imaging privileges or refused to undergo these inspections.[50] A similar program in Massachusetts resulted in 18% of nonradiologist physicians ceasing to bill payers, without undergoing site inspection.[22] Although privileging programs in imaging have never been legislated at the state or federal level, the implementation of these programs by payers, in addition to the CMS mandate for accreditation, can help substantially curb self-referral.

Certificate of Need Legislation

Certificate of need (CON) laws exist in many states, requiring state approval before installation of particular types of equipment costing more than a given threshold within hospitals or private facilities. These laws can make it more difficult for self-referring physicians to enter the practice of imaging, but can also limit the opportunities for hospitals and radiologists to expand imaging practices. Although the previously described limitations on imaging privileges and audit provisions can be initiated by payers, CON legislation remains the purview of state governments.

SUMMARY

Turf battles present complex challenges, beginning with delineation of turf. In fact, drawing boundaries around quality, measured as accuracy of interpretation, adherence to accreditation standards, and evaluation of outcomes, may make more sense than mere border patrol against invasion. This article focuses on being a caretaker of turf and, in medical practice, its inhabitants: the patients. This movement represents an important shift in focus from being obsessed with landowner status. Complicating the issue further, quality must be realized while cost is controlled. This objective can be achieved through addressing overuse, which in turn requires confronting the issue of self-referral, both major contributing factors to turf battles. The concept presented is to rely on privileging and accreditation mechanisms and appropriateness criteria (all ideally connected to reimbursement policy) to control the borders, and eliminate the weeds. Keeping patients central to the discussion is not only critical but an obligation of the radiology profession. Mutually beneficial is its impact on turf maintenance, keeping the radiologist relevant and valuable to clinical medicine. Further fulfilling the professional commitment requires setting and keeping high training standards and practice guidelines. Emphasis on subspecialty clinical expertise, pathology correlation, and consideration of the molecular level is important. A multidisciplinary effort in the last two dimensions, training standards and practice guidelines, will serve to build bridges to adjacent turf rather than isolating the profession's own, surrounded by a moat. Active participation in high-level research will ensure that radiology leads the way in the development and application of advanced imaging modalities and techniques. Finally, no other physician specialty is better equipped, in terms of training and experience, to ensure both quality and patient safety while advancing imaging science.

Turf battles have been described as "vexing, fractious, frustrating, and often nebulous."[46] However, even in the setting of subspecialty crossfire,[51] radiology can both survive and succeed. Following the advice of W.M. Gilmore, almost three-quarters of a century ago, *"We must not forget we are, first, physicians, secondly, radiologists."*[52]

REFERENCES

1. Levin DC, Rao VM. Turf wars in radiology: introduction. J Am Coll Radiol 2004;1:23–5.
2. Dorfman GS. Can we learn lessons from history or are we condemned to repeat it? Invest Radiol 1994;29:485–8.
3. Judkins MP. Selective coronary angiography: IA percutaneous transfemoral technique. Radiology 1967;89:815–24.
4. Amplatz K, Formanek G, Stanger P, et al. Mechanics of selective coronary artery catheterization via femoral approach. Radiology 1967;89:1040–7.
5. Levin DC, Abrams HL, Castaneda-Zuniga WR, et al. Lessons from history: Why radiologists lost coronary angiography, and what can be done to prevent future similar losses. Invest Radiol 1994;29:480–4.
6. The Balanced Budget Act of 1997. Pub L No. 105-33, 111 Stat 251 (Aug. 5, 1997).
7. Levin DC, Rao VM. Turf wars in radiology: the overutilization of imaging resulting from self-referral. J Am Coll Radiol 2004;1:169–72.
8. Hillman BJ, Joseph CA, Mabry MR, et al. Frequency and costs of diagnostic imaging in office practice— a comparison of self-referring and radiologist-referring physicians. N Engl J Med 1990;323:1604–8.
9. Hillman BJ, Olson GT, Griffith PE, et al. Physician's utilization and charges for outpatient diagnostic imaging in a Medicare population. JAMA 1992; 268:2050–4.
10. Referrals to physician-owned imaging facilities warrant HCFA's scrutiny. report to the Chairman, Subcommittee on Health, Committee on Ways and Means, House of Representatives. GAO/HEHS-95–2. Washington, DC: U.S. General Accounting Office; 1994.
11. Maloney MC, Grajower MM, Burris JF, et al. Frequency and cost of diagnostic imaging in office practice— a comparison of self-referring and radiologist-referring physicians [Letters]. N Engl J Med 1991; 324:1371–2.
12. Alagona P Jr, Cooley DA, Varipapa RJ. Physicians and outpatient diagnostic imaging: overexposed? [Letters]. JAMA 1993;269:1633.
13. Baumgarten DA, Nelson RC. Outcomes of examinations self-referred as a result of spiral CT of the abdomen. Acad Radiol 1997;4:802–5.
14. Levin DC, Rao VM. Turf wars in radiology: other causes of overutilization and what can be done about it. J Am Coll Radiol 2004;1:317–21.
15. Levin DC, Rao VM. Turf wars in radiology: the quality of interpretations of imaging studies by nonradiologist physicians—a patient safety issue? J Am Coll Radiol 2004;1:506–9.
16. Potchen EJ, Cooper TG, Sierra AE, et al. Measuring performance in chest radiography. Radiology 2000; 217:456–9.
17. Eng J, Mysko WK, Weller GER, et al. Interpretation of emergency department radiographs: a comparison of emergency medicine physicians with radiologists, residents with faculty, and film with digital display. Am J Roentgenol 2000;175:1233–8.
18. Alfaro D, Levitt MA, English DK, et al. Accuracy of interpretation of cranial computed tomography scans in an emergency medicine residency program. Ann Emerg Med 1995;25:169–74.
19. Kohn LT, Corrigan JM, Donaldson MS. To err is human: building a safer health system. Washington, DC: National Academy Press; 2000.
20. Tieman J. Study finds care quality lacking. Mod Healthc 2002;32:24.
21. Edmiston RB, Levin DC. Film quality assessment varies among specialties. Diagn Imaging (San Franc) 1992;14:37–9.
22. Verrilli DK, Bloch SM, Rousseau J, et al. Design of a privileging program for diagnostic imaging: costs and implications for a large insurer in Massachusetts. Radiology 1998;208:385–92.
23. Levin DC, Rao VM, Orrison WW. Turf wars in radiology: the quality of imaging facilities operated by non-radiologist physicians and of the images they produce. J Am Coll Radiol 2004;1:649–51.
24. The Medicare Improvements for Patients and Providers Act of 2008. Pub L No. 110-275, 122 Stat 2494 (July 15, 2008).
25. Rao VM, Levin DC. Turf wars in radiology: training in diagnostic imaging: How much is enough? J Am Coll Radiol 2005;2:1016–8.

26. Rao VM, Levin DC. Turf wars in radiology: the past, present and future importance of training standards in imaging. J Am Coll Radiol 2005;2:602–6.

27. Medicare Payment Advisory Commission. Report to the Congress: Medicare payment policy. Available at: http://www.medpac.gov/publications/congressional_reports/mar05_ch03.pdf.

28. Borgstede JP. The viability of our specialty: the designated physician imager. J Am Coll Radiol 2005;2:99–102.

29. Wechsler RJ, Spettell CM, Kurtz AB, et al. Effects of training and experience in interpretation of emergency body CT scans. Radiology 1996;199: 717–20.

30. Hertzberg BS, Kliewer MS, Bowie JD, et al. Physician training requirements in sonography: how many cases are needed for competence? Am J Roentgenol 2000;174:1221–7.

31. Weinreb JC, Wilcox PA. How do training, education, and experience affect quality in radiology? J Am Coll Radiol 2004;1:510–5.

32. Gollub MJ, Panicek DM, Bach AM, et al. Clinical importance of reinterpretations of body CT scans obtained elsewhere in patients referred for care at a tertiary cancer center. Radiology 1999;210: 109–12.

33. Dudley RA, Hricak H, Scheidler, et al. Shared patient analysis. A method to assess the clinical benefits of patient referrals. Med Care 2001;39:1182–7.

34. Guiberteau MJ. 2006 ACR Presidential Oration, The ring in the radiograph: profession and principle. J Am Coll Radiol 2007;4:11–7.

35. Levin DC, Rao VM, Bree RL, et al. Turf battles in radiology: how the radiology community can collectively respond to the challenge. Radiology 1999;211: 301–5.

36. Levin DC, Rao VM. Turf wars in radiology: possible remedies for self-referral that could be taken by federal or state governments and payers. J Am Coll Radiol 2004;1:806–10.

37. Babiarz LS, Yousem DM, Parker P, et al. Volume of neuroradiology studies read by neurologists:

implications for fellowship training. J Am Coll Radiol 2011;8:477–82.

38. Levin DC, Rao VM. Turf wars in radiology: updated evidence on the relationship between self-referral and the overutilization of imaging. J Am Coll Radiol 2008;5:806–10.

39. Program requirements for residency education in diagnostic radiology. In: Graduate medical education directory, 1998-1999. Chicago: American Medical Association; 1998. p. 293–6.

40. Rao VM, Levin DC. Turf wars in radiology: what must Academic radiology do? J Am Coll Radiol 2007;4: 622–5.

41. Lillard A. Turf War? Imaging Economics. Available at: http://www.highbeam.com.

42. Paz D. The radiologist as a physician consultant. J Am Coll Radiol 2010;7(9):664–6.

43. American college of radiology. ACR appropriateness criteria. Radiology 2000;215(Suppl):1–1511.

44. Hillman BJ. Doing well by doing good: the ACRIN fund for imaging innovation. J Am Coll Radiol 2006;3:307–8.

45. Hillman BJ. Isn't anybody paying attention? J Am Coll Radiol 2004;1:302–3.

46. Levin DC, Rao VM. Turf wars in radiology: the future of Radiology depends on research-and your support of it! J Am Coll Radiol 2007;4:184–6.

47. Borgstede JP. Strategies for the future. J Am Coll Radiol 2006;3:305–6.

48. Levin DC. The practice of radiology by nonradiologists: cost, quality, and utilization issues. Am J Roentgenol 1994;162:513–8.

49. Hillman BJ. Self-referral for diagnostic imaging. Radiology 1992;185:633–4.

50. Moskowitz H, Sunshine J, Grossman D, et al. The effect of imaging guidelines on the number and quality of outpatient radiographic examinations. Am J Roentgenol 2000;175:9–15.

51. Patoine B. Neuroimaging turf battles flare. Ann Neurol 2008;A13–6.

52. Gilmore WM. The radiologist as a consultant. CMAJ 1940;42:357–60.

The Resource-Based Relative Value Scale and Neuroradiology
ASNR's History at the RUC

William D. Donovan, MD, MPH

KEYWORDS

- Resource-based relative value scale • American Medical Association/Specialty Society RVS Update Committee • Medicare • American Society of Neuroradiology
- Centers for Medicare and Medicaid Services

KEY POINTS

- The Resource-Based Relative Value Scale (RBRVS), the foundation of physician professional payment in the United States, was established in 1992.
- Radiology had already established its own relative value scale (RVS), which was wholly incorporated into the RBRVS.
- The American Society of Neuroradiology first participated in the American Medical Association/Specialty Society RVS Update Committee (RUC) process in 1998, and has been actively engaged since then.
- In recent years the RUC, Centers for Medicare and Medicaid Services, and the Medicare Payment Advisory Committee have squarely targeted radiology procedures for diminished valuation on multiple fronts.

INTRODUCTION

Before 1992, professional payment for Medicare services in the United States was fragmented, usually administered on a local or regional basis. There was significant geographic variation in reimbursement of doctors' fees. With health care cost outlays accelerating rapidly in the 1980s, there was a call by Congress for greater oversight of distribution of government revenue for medical services. This led to the creation of the Resource-Based Relative Value Scale (RBRVS), which remains in force, with continual evolution, to the current day. The radiology community played a critical role, perhaps more than any other single medical specialty, in the acceptance of the relative value scale (RVS) system by the greater medical community. The neuroradiology community, despite its small numeric footprint nationwide, has participated actively in the evolution of this payment system.

BRIEF HISTORY OF THE RBRVS

The Medicare program was created by the Social Security Act of 1965, signed into law by then-President Lyndon B. Johnson (Fig. 1). It reimbursed physicians for both their professional work and their direct practice expenses on an as-billed basis. There was a modest oversight program to confirm that reimbursement requests were in line with "customary, prevailing, and

Disclosures: None.
Department of Diagnostic Imaging, The William W. Backus Hospital, 326 Washington Street, Norwich, CT 06360, USA
E-mail address: william.donovan@snet.net

Neuroimag Clin N Am 22 (2012) 421–436
doi:10.1016/j.nic.2012.04.008

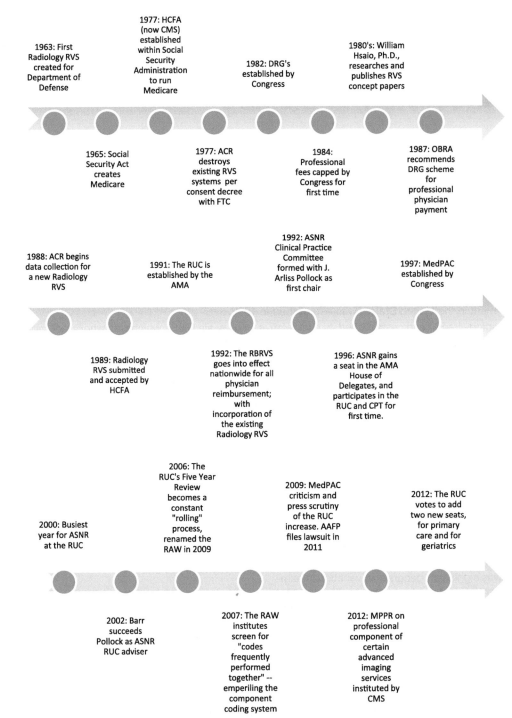

Fig. 1. Timeline of the Resource-Based Relative Value Scale. AAFP, American Academy of Family Physicians; ACR, American College of Radiology; AMA, American Medical Association; ASNR, American Society of Neuroradiology; CMS, Centers for Medicare and Medicaid Services; CPT, Current Procedural Terminology; DRG, Diagnosis-Related Group; FTC, Federal Trade Commission; HCFA, Health Care Financing Administration; MedPAC, Medicare Payment Advisory Committee; MPPR, Multiple Procedure Percent Reduction; OBRA, Omnibus Budget Reconciliation Act; RAW, Relativity Assessment Workgroup; RUC, American Medical Association/Specialty Society RVS Update Committee; RVS, Relative Value Scale.

reasonable" charges, but no organized national basis or guidelines to maintain uniformity. The Health Care Financing Administration (HCFA) was established in 1977 as a separate administrative entity within the Social Security Administration to run Medicare (HCFA was renamed the Centers for Medicare and Medicaid Services [CMS] in 2001).

This nonuniform scheme of reimbursement remained in force with minimal alteration into the 1980s. The 1982 Tax Equity and Fiscal Responsibility Act was passed into law partly in response to the burgeoning federal monetary outlays that occurred in the 1970s.[1] It established the Diagnosis-Related Group (DRG) system for payment of inpatient medical expenses: hospitals were subsequently paid an established fee for the cost of inpatient care based on specific diagnosis or diagnoses attributed to the patient. These fixed amounts were calculated by averaging actual hospital costs prior to that time. The legislation achieved its desired effect: inpatient costs to Medicare stabilized. There was a measurable decrease in inpatient days, and a shift to preferential outpatient care of medical illness and surgery.[2]

This system also solidified a separation of physicians' payments (which were not directly addressed by the DRG legislation) and hospital payments. Already in process, this program accelerated the increased prevalence of radiologists detaching themselves from hospital employment, with increased establishment of professional corporations that contracted with hospitals and maintained separate billing arrangements; in this way they untied themselves from the DRG model.[1] This is also manifested by the separation of professional fees for interpretation of imaging studies from technical fees, the performance of the studies.

With the success of the DRG model at controlling hospital-based costs, then about two-thirds of Medicare's budget, there was subsequently a call for control of physician payments. In 1984, professional reimbursement to physicians was frozen, at first for 1 year, then extended to a second. Physician charges to Medicare patients were also capped, limiting the previous custom of "balance-billing" beyond the maximum government payments. Attention was also directed toward perceived nationwide inequities in physician payment, both geographically and between specialists and primary care providers.

In an effort to control, monitor, and regulate physician payments, Congress commissioned William Hsiao, PhD, of the Harvard School of Public Health, to establish a "relative value scale" (RVS) for professional payment. In a series of research articles in the 1980s, he had proposed and justified such a system, and had become a national spokesperson in this concept.[3,4]

An RVS is a means of estimating the discrete amount of work that goes into providing a specific medical service in relation to other procedures; that is, to create a schedule or table that ranks procedures in order. To do this, the concept of "physician work" first needed to be defined. Hsiao's system did this by estimating the amount of time a procedure required, and the difficulty or intensity of the procedure. Intensity was defined by 3 subcategories: technical skill or physical effort; mental effort or judgment; and stress. The latter concept of psychological stress was used as a surrogate for the possibility of being subjected to a lawsuit in the event of an untoward outcome. Thus procedures that took a long time, but which were easier to perform and less likely to lead to a malpractice action, might be valued less than a procedure requiring less time but which was more intense, challenging, and stressful. The essential technique by which Hsiao had physicians estimate their work was a statistical concept of "magnitude estimation": by simply asking a sufficient number of physicians how they would rank a list of procedures from the least amount of work to the greatest (while keeping in mind the 3 metrics listed above), a statistically reliable and reproducible means of creating an RVS was established. In addition, Hsiao acknowledged and incorporated the concept that practice expenses were an essential ingredient in physician reimbursement.[3]

THE ROLE OF RADIOLOGY IN THE ADOPTION OF THE RVS

Less well known than Hsiao's arrival on the national payment scene is the key role played by the radiology community in the adoption of the RVS system. Radiology's efforts to establish an RVS actually predated Hsiao; and during the 1980s, radiology's RVSs were being revised and updated contemporaneous with Hsiao's efforts.

Radiology initially established an RVS of its own as early as 1963 in response to a request from the Department of Defense for its own insurance program for military and dependents. In 1965, the American College of Radiology (ACR) revised this initial charge-based scale to base its system on "time and effort devoted by the radiologist."[1] Additional revisions followed in 1969 and 1973, the latter including practice expenses incurred for each procedure. There was a temporary moratorium on development and promulgation of RVSs in the mid-1970s resulting from a decree by the Federal Trade Commission that such systems were anticompetitive. All previously established

RVSs were actually deleted by the ACR.[1] However, when the legislative tide turned back toward the use of RVSs in the 1980s, the ACR's previous work in this area was resurrected.

The Omnibus Budget Reconciliation Act of 1987 (OBRA1987), based on the success of the earlier cost-control efforts detailed above, included multiple provisions that we now recognize as inherent to the health care payment system in the United States: budget neutrality, with establishment of an annually adjusted conversion factor; allowance for scheduled geographic variation in costs; further limitations on (and ultimately proscription of) balance-billing above the allowed Medicare charges; and that such an RVS would be created in collaboration with provider stakeholders (for instance the ACR) and legislative review.[5] The latter was enabled by the newly formed Physician Payment Review Commission (PPRC), an advisory body made up largely of physicians, whose stamp of approval significantly facilitated Congressional action.[6] However, OBRA1987 contained another provision that galvanized the radiology community: rather than wait for Hsaio's RVS work to be completed, it directed the HCFA to develop DRGs for payment of hospital-based specialty physicians (radiology, anesthesia, and pathology), and directed that such a system be adopted for the 1989 Federal Budget.

The threat of Federal government fee-setting for radiology services was acted on swiftly and effectively by the ACR. In addition to a presumed decrease in professional revenue, there was the strong likelihood that hospitals would again become the dominant employer of radiologists under such a system.[1] In congressional testimony, the ACR volunteered to work with Congress, the HCFA, and the PPRC to develop an alternative means of reimbursing radiologists that would be acceptable to Washington. In consultation with the PPRC and the HCFA, and based on its earlier experience, the ACR created a new radiology RVS. Magnitude estimation data (in the form of surveys of 45 radiology services) were collected; these data was refined by consensus of expert panels of radiologists; and then extrapolated to include every radiology service then described (numbering 740) in the Current Procedural Terminology (CPT) guidebook of the American Medical Association (AMA). One hundred ten other services outside the radiology section, but also commonly performed by radiologists, were also ranked. The data collection specifically requested information on the key concepts described above: the time required for a service; and physician effort, including the subcategories of technical skill or physical effort, mental effort or judgment, and

stress. This overall assessment of physician work was termed "complexity," and some of the parameters measured by Hsaio were rephrased (component dimensions included time, mental effort, technical skill, quality control and assurance, and potential harm to patient).

Two thousand work surveys were sent out to practicing radiologists in 1988; 1022 responses were received. Three thousand surveys on professional and global charges were sent; almost 1800 were received. Data on practice expense were collected by an independent professional consulting group from 400 practices nationwide. The results were subsequently analyzed by ACR subcommittees of diverse background and subspecialty. The intravenous pyelogram was chosen as the key reference procedure for the entire spectrum, and set at an arbitrary nonmonetary value of 100. With the survey results of the 45 "primary" services in hand, and with the advice of the subspecialty committees, the ACR's steering committee established an RVS for more than 800 procedures by magnitude estimation in a matter of months through numerous meetings and conference calls.[1] The sheer size of this data collection and analysis, especially in view of the pencil-and-paper nature of the surveys, and the compressed time frame in which it occurred, remains an achievement of staggering proportions to this day. Based on the compelling strength of the work performed by the ACR, the HCFA accepted the submitted recommendations for professional relative work values in radiology for the 1989 budget without change, predating the HCFA's adoption of Hsaio's system for the rest of medicine by 3 years.[7] The only amendment was that the HCFA declined to accept ACR's recommendations for those procedures outside the Radiology section of the CPT guidebook.

The HCFA instituted the so-called RBRVS for the entire Medicare fee schedule, phased-in between 1992 and 1996, based mostly on Hsaio's work. Hsaio's RBRVS adopted the radiology RVS in toto, without adjustment, which is further testimony to the statistical strength of the ACR effort.[7] Besides establishing reliable reimbursement schedules for Medicare patients, many private payors use the Medicare fee schedule as a basis for their own, emphasizing its critical role.

THE RISE OF COMPONENT CODING

In the establishment of the radiology RVS, and the nascent establishment of the national RBRVS for Medicare, local discrepancies in the coding of interventional procedures were uncovered. Specifically, some Medicare carriers reimbursed interventional procedures in a bundled manner, whereas the radiology RVS and the ACR advocated billing on a component basis; that is, separate codes for supervision and radiologic interpretation (S and I) of interventional procedures apart from the billing of the surgical procedure itself. Further, some carriers would reimburse for a complete surgical procedure as if a single procedure had been performed, whereas others reimbursed separately for the discrete building blocks of the entire surgical portion of an interventional procedure. The ACR was insistent that the latter component-based system was appropriate, both for more accurate reimbursement and for better tracking of procedures for quality control, practice expense, and trend analysis. Through dedicated efforts on the part of ACR and the Society of Interventional Radiology (SIR) (then the Society of Cardiovascular and Interventional Radiology), in the form of numerous negotiations and proposals with the HCFA, a nationwide standardized approach of component coding and reimbursement was adopted into the radiology RVS in 1991, and subsequently incorporated into the RBRVS.[1]

THE RUC

One of PPAC's recommendations to Congress made during consideration of a national Medicare RBRVS was to establish an expert multispecialty consensus panel that would be charged with ongoing review of the accuracy of the RBRVS, and that would determine appropriate rank-order placement of newly introduced procedures into the system.[8] Thus was born the RUC, an acronym for the American Medical Association/Specialty Society RVS Update Committee, which continues its work on an advisory basis to CMS to the present day. The RUC first met in May 1991. As further evidence of the respect with which ACR's process was regarded, the nascent RUC sought advice and input from the ACR on its successful survey model.[1]

During the thrice-yearly RUC meetings, advisors from medical specialty societies (now more than 100) present recommendations to the Committee regarding their assessment of the relative value of procedures performed by its members. The Committee currently consists of 29 members, 23 of whom are physicians nominated by the major specialty societies (Box 1).[9,10] Radiology holds a seat on the Committee, and the ACR nominates a Member who serves upon the approval of the AMA. The other radiology societies regularly in attendance at RUC meetings are the American Society of Neuroradiology (ASNR) and SIR. The Society of Nuclear Medicine (SNM) also attends

faithfully. The representatives of these societies have formed a close working bond over the years, persevering through occasional changes in personnel.

The process of the RUC meeting has evolved over the past 20 years, but its mission has remained focused: to cogently place a procedure in its appropriate place in the hierarchy of professional medical work by assigning a defensible relative value unit (RVU) value. The values suggested by the societies are debated, and frequently revised by the Committee. The RVU values decided on by the RUC are then passed along to the CMS, who may adopt these values, or change them to their liking, before incorporating them into the Medicare Physician Fee Schedule (PFS). The RUC has been, and remains, the primary advisory body supplying information and recommendations to CMS for professional work valuation and practice expense (Fig. 2).

In the 20 years of its existence, the RUC has provided a very effective service to CMS. More than 90% of its RVU recommendations have been accepted by the CMS in its annual PFS.[10] This track record stalled somewhat in 2011, when the CMS accepted just 85% of the RUC's recommendations, revaluing the other 15% in its Proposed and Final Rules.

Societies develop their recommendations to the RUC by means of standardized surveys that are sent to their membership. The physician completing the survey is asked to assess the amount of time a procedure takes; how it ranks in terms of work compared with a list of comparable procedures provided by the specialty; and to compare the procedure in question with the most commonly chosen reference service for "intensity and complexity." These questions ask the responder to quantify the technical skill, physical difficulty, and mental stress of the examination.

One of the key elements of the RUC process is the concept of budget neutrality: increasing the RVU value of one procedure in a zero-sum system will lead to less reimbursement for all other procedures. There is an obvious incentive to achieve maximal achievable RVU values for codes that one's own society members perform, and to critique (where possible) other societies' attempts to maximize their code values. This potentially antagonistic situation is tempered by the frequent need for cooperation between societies to present codes together in frequently shifting alliances. Furthermore, voting members of the RUC itself are specifically barred from advocating for code valuations presented by the societies they represent; they are charged with sitting as impartial judges of valuation. These checks and balances tend to dampen intersocietal conflict.

Box 1
Composition of the RUC

Chair

American Medical Association Representative

CPT Editorial Panel Representative

American Osteopathic Association Representative

Health Care Professionals Advisory Committee Representative

Practice Expense Subcommittee Representative

Anesthesiology

Cardiology

Cardiothoracic surgery

Dermatology

Emergency Medicine

Family medicine

General surgery

Internal medicine

Neurology

Neurosurgery

Obstetrics/gynecology

Ophthalmology

Orthopedic surgery

Otolaryngology

Pathology

Pediatrics

Plastic surgery

Psychiatry

Radiology

Urology

Infectious Disease

Rheumatology[a]

Vascular surgery[a]

Primary care[b]

Geriatrics[b]

[a] Rotating seat: not specifically designated for those specialties.
[b] Added in 2012.
  Data from American Medical Association. 2012 RVS Update Process. Available at: http://www.ama-assn.org/resources/doc/rbrvs/ruc-update-booklet.pdf.

THE ASNR AT THE RUC

The ASNR was founded in 1962.[11] Throughout its history, the mission of the Society was focused on education and dissemination of information to its members, and to the rest of the medical community.[12] An emphasis on socioeconomic and political activity in the ASNR beginning in the 1990s is directly attributable to the work of one man: J. Arliss Pollock, MD (Fig. 3).

Arliss Pollock was a native of Texas. After 4 years of military service, he completed a radiology residency and a fellowship in neuroradiology at the University of California, San Francisco. In 1967, he joined a private practice group, Radiological Associates in Sacramento, as the first neuroradiologist

The CPT – RUC Process Cycle

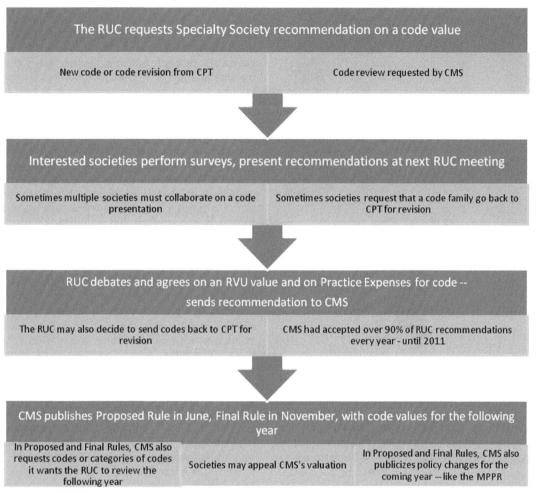

Fig. 2. The CPT-RUC process cycle.

in that city. He was instrumental in bringing the first computed tomography (CT) and magnetic resonance (MR) imaging scanners to a private practice environment in that area. He was renowned as a skilled neuroradiologist in both diagnostic and catheter-based procedures. He received a "Golden Stethoscope" award from the Sacramento-Yolo County Medical Society in 1989 as its outstanding physician of the year (of any specialty). He was a founding member of the Western Neuroradiological Society, and served as its president. He coauthored several scholarly articles, still cited, related to catheter angiography technique, quality control, and patient safety.[13–15] In 2001 he was awarded the ASNR Gold Medal, the highest honor the Society bestows, citing his promotion of "the recognition of neuroradiology to government agencies and other medical societies to develop and strengthen our presence and effectiveness at the national and state levels" through the development

of "a broad strategy of activities to participate as a society not previously within our mission."[16,17]

His work in the sphere of socioeconomic policy at ASNR has become legendary. "I can tell you that without Arliss, there would have been no focus of ASNR on socioeconomic issues in the early 90s," according to ASNR past-president Eric J. Russell, MD; "Arliss had a command of the issues second to no one" (Russell EJ, personal communication, 2012). He served as the founding chairman of the Clinical Practice Committee (CPC) from 1992 until 2004. The purpose of that committee was and is to provide ASNR membership with a political voice and presence, to assist membership with reimbursement issues, and to help provide justification for their services in a practical manner; that is, integrating research, use, standards, and quality activities with active clinical practice. Through the CPC, he focused on promulgation of the Society's presence on the national

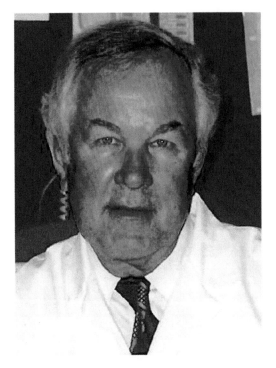

Fig. 3. J. Arliss Pollock, MD.

medical scene. He spearheaded efforts within the Society to gain recognition from the AMA in the form of a delegate seat, by promoting AMA membership amongst ASNR members.[18] The AMA has only allowed specialty societies to attend and participate in AMA House of Delegate meetings, and in CPT and RUC meetings, if a certain percentage of their membership joins the AMA (this percentage has changed over the years). This effort led by Dr Pollock was met with success in 1996, with the establishment of a delegate seat in the AMA; this allowed ASNR to send advisors to the RUC, and to CPT Panel meetings. Pollock expanded his service to the Society by becoming its first advisor to the RUC. He served in this capacity until 2002.

Dr Pollock stressed the importance of national payment policy in the consciousness of ASNR members, and ensured the recognition of neuroradiology on the national medical scene. He recognized that involvement in the CPT and RUC process was integral to the subspecialty's success. As described in earlier sections, the AMA has managed to define medical practice in North America in a basic yet pervasive numerical manner through its copyright of the CPT guidebook and coding system, and to thereby influence professional physician reimbursement through the advisory capacity of the RUC. Pollock realized in his early years of ASNR involvement that the

specialty of neuroradiology deserved the opportunity to participate in the specific and detailed defining of medical procedures (in the CPT process), and in their valuation (at the RUC), in a manner that would earn neuroradiology increased respect and recognition from their medical and surgical colleagues, as well as from the medical device and equipment industries. This appreciation for the complex aspects of payment policy coincided with that of another radiologist in Sacramento, James M. Moorefield, MD, who had spearheaded the adoption of the Radiology RVS into the RBRVS and who represented Radiology on the RUC in the 1990s. According to Dr Moorefield, Pollock needed no encouragement to throw himself into the payment policy arena: "he came ready to fight, and advocated for neuroradiology in a tireless and very effective manner" (Moorefield JM, personal communication, 2012).

To further the legitimacy of neuroradiologists' work, Pollock formulated the subcommittee structure of the CPC to focus on the scientific foundation for the economics work that he and other ASNR members were doing at the national level. In addition to a subcommittee focused on CPT/RUC Committee work, he also established subcommittees of Practice Guidelines and Technical Standards; Appropriateness Criteria, Utilization, and Quality; and Governmental Affairs. By providing a foundation on safe and effective practice that could be documented and demonstrated to the medical community, he was able to emphasize the legitimacy, safety, and efficacy of neurointerventional procedures, CT, and MR imaging. These efforts provided the groundwork for establishment and revision of multiple CPT codes with direct neuroradiologist input. These codes were then brought to the RUC by Pollock himself (and by his successors) for RVU valuation. His quiet enthusiasm on behalf of the subspecialty was rewarded in a very practical sense: reimbursement for many specific neuroradiologic procedures is directly attributable to Pollock's efforts.

A prominent example of his involvement in the codification and valuation of a previously unlisted procedure is vertebroplasty, for which 6 separately reportable codes were created and valued in the year 2000. It should be noted that this was a multisociety effort, requiring close collaboration with the ACR and SIR, and neurosurgery societies, as well as with the pioneering efforts of Dr Mary E. Jensen in the CPT process.

He collaborated closely with a collection of other nonradiology societies (mostly spine and pain management groups) on numerous injection codes (epidural injections, transforaminal injections, facet injections), with successful maintenance of component coding, and separate reporting of radiologic supervision and interpretation.

2000 was a banner year for ASNR at the RUC. In addition to participating in vetebroplasty evaluation, Dr Pollock also presented 6 new codes for MR angiography of the head and of the neck in April 2000. MR angiography examinations of the head and neck before 2000 had a single code designation, no matter how simply or elaborately it was performed in a given instance. Pollock (along with ASNR staff, ACR staff, and advisors) established 6 separate CPT codes for MR angiographic examinations of the head and of the neck, with the various permutations for studies performed with intravenous contrast, without contrast, and both, and securing favorable RVU valuations that have survived to this day. He also managed to guide codes for contrast-enhanced MR imaging of the head and neck (orbit/face/neck, in CPT terminology) through the RUC in 2000, and managed to do so without being required to resurvey the membership for the noncontrast base code, the valuation of which has survived from 1992. Pollock and ACR colleagues also brought forward separate CT angiography codes for the head and for the neck that year, which he presented and which were appropriately valued through ASNR and ACR teamwork.

During his CPC chairmanship and RUC advisor years, he also pursued CPT recognition and RUC valuation for other multiple other procedures as diverse as CT perfusion of the head, temporary balloon occlusion, MR spectroscopy, and magnetoencephalography.[19] He worked intensely on developing code descriptions for functional MR imaging. Although that family of codes was not valued until after his time at the RUC, he was instrumental in diplomatically maintaining ASNR's prominence in the debate over CPT wording and work descriptors, when faced with representatives from other societies who questioned the central role of radiology in these procedures (Barr RM, personal communication).

According to Dr Robert M. Barr, Pollock's successor as RUC advisor and current chair of the CPC, "[Arliss] was very diplomatic and polished at the RUC. He was bold when he felt action was needed...but he also knew when to stay out of the way" (Barr RM, personal communication, 2012). This synopsis reflects a grasp of the sometimes delicate balance that societies, especially subspecialty societies, must tread at RUC meetings and in the preparations leading to those meetings. Many radiology and neuroradiology procedures values were adopted into the RBRVS in 1992 with the Radiology RVS, and have had so-

called Harvard valuation, reflecting Hsaio's base of operations. Many of these values have been maintained through the years (until recently), at least partly on the strength of the Radiology RVS survey process. Another sizeable group of radiology codes have had the designation of "CMS/Other"; this group was adopted into the RVS, then had their values affirmed at the First Five-Year Review (5YR) in 1995. Codes included in these groups include brain and spine MR imaging, head CT, facial bone CT, neck CT, carotid angiography codes, and codes for positron emission tomography of the brain. One of the unwritten duties of the RUC advisory teams from ASNR, ACR, and SIR through the years has been to ensure as much as possible that "historically valued" procedures such as these stayed out of the limelight; for instance, by not using them as validation for other codes, and by declining to bring them forward to the RUC in an attempt to increase their valuation, a process that can backfire.

An example of this strategy has been the reluctance of ASNR economics team members to request advancement of CT perfusion of the head from a Category III code to a Category I code in the CPT process. (The Category III codes are "temporary" codes, usually applied to new or emerging technology, and not meeting criteria for Category I codes.[20] Category III codes are not valued by the RUC, and are not assigned value by CMS, although third-party payors may reimburse them.) In the recent RUC climate, it has become the norm for the RUC to review any related codes in the "family" of the code brought forward. Thus, it is likely that the RUC would have insisted on a formal survey and reevaluation of the basic head CT codes (70450, 70460, 70470: without contrast, with contrast, and without/with contrast, respectively). These codes had never been through the "modern" RUC survey process; their values were incorporated into the RBRVS from the radiology RVS, and affirmed without survey in the 1995 First 5YR. Although the strength and validity of those old surveys have been affirmed over the years, they are now looked on with skepticism by the RUC because of updates in the survey process that have occurred since. Thus, advancing the CT perfusion code may have put the valuation of the most commonly performed CT examination in the Medicare population at risk. The next sections discuss further where recent RUC initiatives and trends have thrown new light on many of these Harvard-valued and CMS/Other procedures, including the head CT family.

Without the forward thinking and tireless dedication of Dr Pollock, the ASNR could have remained voiceless in the CPT/RUC process, and a significantly more marginal presence in the national radiology and medical payment policy arena. Table 1 lists the volunteer physicians who have served the ASNR at the RUC and at CPT Panel meetings.

ASNR AT THE RUC, 2004 TO THE PRESENT

Dr Patrick A. Turski assumed chairmanship of the ASNR CPC in 2004, serving until 2010. Barr became the ASNR's RUC advisor in 2002, serving until 2008 (see Table 1). He has recently assumed chairmanship of the CPC. These individuals have continued the active presence in matters of payment policy, quality assurance, appropriateness and standards, and intersocietal activity that Dr Pollock established. The Government Affair subcommittee was folded into the ACR Neuroradiology Commission during Dr Turski's era, in an effort to align these matters with the ACR's Governmental Affairs activities.

The ASNR spearheaded or participated in the introduction of numerous new procedures through the CPT and RUC process during this decade, including intraoperative MR imaging (2003); kyphoplasty (2005); intracranial angioplasty and stenting (2005); carotid stenting (2005); and functional MR imaging (2006) (Table 2). CPT validation and RUC review of these new technologies required concerted efforts on the part of ASNR advisors and staff in multiple channels: collation

of research studies demonstrating their effectiveness; preparation, dissemination, and analysis of RVU surveys, to gather information to assess the amount of physician work involved; and of course, the actual presentation of data and proposals to the CPT Panel and to the RUC. In each case, cooperation with other societies' advisors and staff was valuable in presenting cogent and unified presentations. Barr's leadership of the RUC process was rewarded with valuations appropriately placed within the rank order of the radiology and surgical procedural databases.

RADIOLOGY IN THE CROSSHAIRS

Evolutionary changes at the RUC over the past 5 years, however, have caused the ASNR and the other radiology societies to assume a more defensive posture.

As one of the founding principles of the RUC, Congress mandated a program to review codes already vetted in an effort to maintain legitimacy and relativity in the face of changing technology and its use. A new technology or procedure, it was assumed, may be more efficiently performed as a physician's experience increases, and/or with equipment improvements. There was also a concern that favorable reimbursement, in the absence of occasional review, could lead to preferential use, inappropriate use, or inappropriate coding.

Table 1
ASNR RUC and CPT advisors and alternates

Year	RUC Advisor	RUC Alternate	CPT Advisor	CPT Alternate
1996–1997	J. Arliss Pollock			
1997–1998	J. Arliss Pollock			
1998–1999	J. Arliss Pollock	Blake A. Johnson	Blake A. Johnson	J. Arliss Pollock
1999–2000	J. Arliss Pollock	Blake A. Johnson	Blake A. Johnson	J. Arliss Pollock
2000–2001	J. Arliss Pollock	Charles M. Citrin	Blake A. Johnson	Mary E. Jensen
2001–2002	J. Arliss Pollock	Charles M. Citrin	Robert A. Murray	Blake A. Johnson
2002–2003	J. Arliss Pollock	Robert M. Barr	Robert A. Murray	Blake A. Johnson
2003–2004	Robert M. Barr	J. Arliss Pollock	Robert A. Murray	
2004–2005	Robert M. Barr	J. Arliss Pollock and Patrick A. Turski	Robert A. Murray	
2005–2006	Robert M. Barr	Patrick A. Turski	Robert A. Murray	
2006–2007	Robert M. Barr	Patrick A. Turski	C. Douglas Phillips	
2007–2008	Robert M. Barr	William D. Donovan	C. Douglas Phillips	
2008–2009	William D. Donovan	Robert M. Barr	C. Douglas Phillips	
2009–2010	William D. Donovan		C. Douglas Phillips	
2010–2011	William D. Donovan		Jacqueline A. Bello	C. Douglas Phillips
2011–2012	Joshua A. Hirsch	Gregory N. Nicola	Jacqueline A. Bello	Raymond K. Tu

Table 2
ASNR participation at the RUC: codes presented or copresented for valuation (grouped by family)

CPT Code	Short Descriptor	RUC Meeting Year
22520–2, 72291–2	Vertebroplasty, Sacroplasty	2000
70496, 70498	CT angiography of head, neck	2000
70542–3	MR imaging orbit/face/neck	2000
70544–9	MR angiography of head, neck	2000
95965–7	Magnetoencephalography	2001
61623	Temporary head and neck vessel occlusion	2002
61624	Permanent transcatheter occlusion CNS	2002
70557–9	Intraoperative brain MR imaging	2003
37215–6, 75960	Percutaneous carotid stent placement	2004
22520–5	Kyphoplasty, Vertebroplasty	2005
61630, 61635	Intracranial angioplasty ± stent	2005
61640–2	Intracranial dilatation vasospasm	2005
22526–7	Intradiscal electrodermal therapy	2006
70554–5, 96020	Functional brain MR imaging, Brain mapping	2006
77003	Fluoroscopic guidance for spine injection	2008
62267	Disc aspiration	2008
64479–95	Facet and intraforaminal epidural injections	2009
72125, 72128, 72131	CT spine (C, T, L) without contrast	2009
76536	Ultrasound exam of head and neck (thyroid)	2009
77003	Fluoroscopic guidance for spine injection	2009
62284	Injection for myelogram	2010
70470	CT head/brain without and with contrast	2011
72100, 72110, 72114, 72120	Radiographic exams of lower spine	2011
36217	Arterial catheterization	2011
72040, 72050, 72052	Radiographic exams of cervical spine	2012
(To be determined)	Craniocervical angiography family	2012

The 5YR process was charged with scrutinizing the RVU database for procedures whose values were thought to need reexamination by stakeholders, including individual societies, CMS, and regional carriers.[7,21] The 4 5YRs completed to date took place in 1995, 2000, 2005, and 2010. According to AMA statistics, the RUC has reviewed values of a total of 3059 codes at the 5YRs, resulting in confirmation of the current values in 1399, an increase in valuation of 1133, and a decrease in valuation of 208. Three hundred nineteen codes were also identified through these reviews that were referred to the CPT Panel for revision or deletion.[22]

Meanwhile, annual increases in health care spending from 1997 through 2008 averaged 6%, more than double the growth rate of the national economy,[23] leading to Congressional and public concerns. In addition to these general budgetary anxieties, there have been protests raised in some circles that there is an unfair disparity in physician pay between specialties or disciplines. The customary refrain is that primary care reimbursement is undervalued, resulting in an undersupply, and a lack of interest by medical students in entering those fields. Critics point to the traditional PFS model as skewed, reimbursing proceduralists preferentially, and without regard to quality of care delivered. Further, many in these camps believe that primary care physicians are underrepresented at the RUC, propagating the cycle onward.[24–27] The AMA has countered these arguments in other publications; one of these states that through many channels, including the establishment of the Evaluation and Management codes, more than 4 billion dollars has been "redistributed" in the physician payment process to primary care specialists. Dr Barbara Levy, current chair of the RUC, and other AMA representatives have been outspoken in their defense of the current system, with arguments including the RUC principle that codes are not evaluated as primary care or proceduralist codes, but on their own merit; and that RUC members are barred from advocating for their own specialty.[28]

In 2006, the Medicare Payment Advisory Committee (MedPAC) declared in its semiannual report to Congress that the RUC's 5YR process was inefficient, and of questionable effectiveness in controlling Medicare costs.[29] MedPAC was established by the Balanced Budget Amendment of 1997 to serve as an advisory body to Congress in the areas of Medicare spending, access to care, and quality of care.[30] Partly in response to this criticism, the CMS subsequently stepped up its scrutiny of physician reimbursement and the RUC process.

With increased CMS involvement in the RUC process, characterized by an increased number of code requests for the RUC to review, the RUC was forced to adapt the 5YR process into an ongoing presence at each RUC meeting, beginning in 2006 (this was termed the rolling 5YR).[31] In recognition that it was no longer an every-5-year phenomenon, the 5YR Identification Workgroup of the RUC was renamed the Relativity Assessment Workgroup (RAW) in 2007. As of the CMS Final Rule for 2012, the "official" 5YR process was retired; the fourth and final 5YR took place in 2010.

CMS has fully engaged in this accelerated review process. In an effort to formalize its requests, it has asked the RUC to examine codes that met various criteria that might indicate "potential misvaluation." Examples of some of these filters, or screens, have included the following: codes demonstrating a significant increase in use; changes in site of service from when a code was originally valued (suggesting a possible evolution in practice expense or technology); codes of low value but high utilization; and codes that still had Harvard valuation (meaning that they have not been reviewed by RUC since the RBRVS was adopted in 1992).

Many of these screens have resulted in a disproportionate number of radiology codes being designated for review by the RAW in comparison with other specialties. Box 2 gives a timeline of one CT code review that has been revised through the RAW process.[32]

THE FALL OF COMPONENT CODING

One of the most perturbing screens that ASNR, ACR, and SIR have been and are still being forced to work through is the "Codes frequently reported together" screen. The rationale for this screen was to identify "physician efficiencies"; that if services are routinely reported together (ie, by the same provider, for the same Medicare beneficiary, on the same day), they effectively represent a single complex service, rather than discrete services, and

that their valuation should reflect these presumed efficiencies. The component coding system incorporated in the original RBRVS, and justified for reasons already described here, had survived until the advent of this screen. But this screen detailing "codes reported together" (initially generated at a congruence of 90%, and subsequently 75%) have repeatedly captured procedures inherent in the component coding structure of interventional procedures, and some body imaging codes as well.

For example, a selective diagnostic angiogram of a right internal carotid artery under the component coding structure would include separate codes for catheterization of a third-order brachiocephalic arterial branch, and the radiologic supervision and interpretation (S&I) of images obtained. If additional images of the intracranial vessels are obtained, an additional S&I code is added. However, the codes for third-order catheterization and angiographic internal carotid S&I have recently been identified in the "codes reported together" screen.

Code pairs meeting the 90% or 75% filters have been placed on the agenda of a joint CPT/RUC workgroup for review, with subsequent revision of entire families that include these procedures into groups of bundled codes at CPT; this is effectively marginalizing the component-coding structure that has heretofore existed. Although individual component codes are in many cases being maintained to provide a means of reporting unusual scenarios, most interventional procedures in the years to come will be reported with significantly fewer and more inclusive codes. This bundling process is under way at press time for carotid angiography and intervention, with CPT and RUC valuation expected for the 2014 PFS cycle. A single procedure code for selective internal carotid angiography will replace the multiple codes described above. This process has already been completed for several peripheral vascular code families, such as for the lower extremities, the renal arteries, and inferior vena cava filter placement. It has also taken place for CT of the abdomen and pelvis, with a particularly arduous valuation process.[33] Bundling of numerous injection codes (facet injections, transforaminal epidural injections, sacroiliac injections) with radiologic S&I has taken place since 2008. In virtually all cases there has been a decrement in professional RVU values for the new combined procedure compared with the summed work of the previous component code structure.

Additional neuroradiology codes at risk of being revised in this fashion include MR angiography of the head and neck, and myelography S&I with the corresponding injection procedure ("surgical") codes. Noncontrast CT of the head and cervical spine,

Box 2
Case in point: the RUC at work

Valuation of 72125: CT of the Cervical Spine Without Contrast

Pre-2009: 1.16 RVU, dating from the 1992 importation of radiology RVS values into the Medicare RBRVS; validated in 1995 at the First 5YR.

July 2008: CMS asks the RUC to examine 114 procedures it terms "fastest growing" (>10% increase in use for Medicare enrollees per year for at least 3 years). Besides 72125, noncontrast CT examinations of the thoracic and lumbar spine, chest, and upper and lower extremities were also designated for review.

October 2008: 72125 and other screened codes are formally identified by the 5YR Identification Work-group (now the Relativity Assessment Workgroup, or RAW) in the "CMS fastest growing" utilization screen. Societies are asked to present action plans for these codes, in effect giving them an opportunity to explain why survey or other review of the current valuation would not be necessary.

February 2009: ASNR/ACR presents its action plan, asserting that the procedure is appropriately valued in rank order, and that survey and RUC review was not necessary. The RAW disagreed, partly because it met the screen mandated by CMS, and partly because it had not been recently surveyed with a "modern" survey instrument (data from the 1992–1995 survey era is not locatable). Survey requested, with presentation at the following RUC meeting.

Summer 2009: Survey performed (along with CT thoracic and lumbar spine surveys). More than 100 ASNR/ACR members respond. Results analyzed, recommendations prepared. Median survey RVU was 1.38. 25th percentile survey value was 1.20.

October 2009: At the RUC meeting, ASNR advisors Barr and Donovan, along with ACR advisor Geraldine McGinty, MD, MBA, and ACR Alternate Advisor Ezequiel Silva III, MD, present their recommendations. This includes a request for an increase in valuation to 1.20 RVU. "Compelling evidence" for an increase in value must be presented and voted on when a request to increase value is made. Factors that ASNR/ACR felt met the "compelling evidence" hurdle included: (a) change in technology since previous valuation (more images, more planes, thinner slices, multiplanar reformats no longer separately billable since deletion of code 76375 in 2006); (b) change in patient population: in 1992 the typical patient would have been an outpatient with radiculopathy; now the typical noncontrast C-spine patient is a trauma patient in an Emergency Room setting, with resultant increase in urgency of decision making and increased liability; and (c) given the change in patient population, there has been a change in the site of service from outpatient to hospital.

Initial RUC review fails to reach consensus, and the code is sent to a Facilitation Committee. The arguments for increase in valuation are made in fuller detail. The Facilitation Committee in a split decision does not agree that an increase in RVU value is warranted, but agrees that the current value is appropriate, and should be maintained.

The full RUC agrees with the findings of the Facilitation Committee, and recommends to CMS maintenance of the current value of 1.16 RVU.

July 2010: CMS Proposed Rule disagrees with the RUC, and proposes a value of 1.0 RVU, with a tangential rationale: "we are concerned [that there may be] bias in the survey results."

Fall–winter 2010: ASNR, ACR, and the AMA (on behalf of the RUC) submit comments in response to the Proposed Rule disagreeing with CMS's down-valuation. (Once the RUC values a code, it will stand up for those values along with the specialty societies involved.) The charge of bias is countered with the argument that the RUC survey instrument is standardized, and that the narrow range of RVU values amongst the reference services in CT will invariably lead to survey values at or close to current values.

January 2011: ACR requests refinement of this value (along with noncontrast CT of the thoracic spine, lumbar spine, and chest). CMS neglects to invite ASNR to participate in the refinement process.

Summer 2011: The CMS Refinement Panel meets by conference call with ACR advisors arguing against CMS's decision.

November 2011: The Final Rule is released, with the RVU value for noncontrast cervical spine CT adjusted upward to 1.07. The values for T-spine and L-spine were not changed at refinement, and remain 1.00. No rationale given in the Final Rule for the varying treatment.

January 1, 2012: The Final Rule value takes effect.

and CT angiography of the head and neck have hovered below the level of "percent-performed-together" deemed actionable by the RAW to date.

It is not yet clear what the effect of the Multiple Procedure Percent Reduction (MPPR) policy applied to professional reimbursement of advanced imaging studies by the 2012 Final Rule will have on this RAW initiative[34]; most advanced imaging code pairs are now subject to an MPPR discount, the bundling of codes frequently performed together seems doubly penalizing (advanced imaging services was defined in the Final Rule as including CT, MR imaging, and ultrasonography). This issue has not yet been directly addressed by the RUC, although the AMA did submit comments to the CMS opposing creation of the MPPR on the professional component.

Not content to suggest filters for the RAW to process, CMS in its Final Rule for 2012 also published its own list of "high-volume, high-expenditure" codes (known in the 2012 Proposed and Final Rules as "Table 7") for which it has requested RUC review. Included in this list are CT of the head and MR imaging of the brain and spine, procedures that to date had evaded 5YR/RAW screens. As already mentioned for head CT, most of the MR imaging codes also have CMS/Other valuations dating from the early 1990s. ASNR action on these codes has already begun, with some being presented at the October 2012 RUC meeting.

ASNR and the other radiology societies are thus engaged on multiple fronts, owing to the substantial numbers of codes identified on multiple screens. At the September 2011 RUC meeting, the radiology societies together were preparing surveys and action plans on over 45 codes. This work pace has not slowed in early 2012, with the ACR, ASNR, and SIR collaborating on about 40 codes under review, in one stage or another, for both January and April meetings.

The RUC and CMS have also expanded its charge to the radiology societies to include the following additional analyses: mandatory practice expense review in conjunction with any physician work review (frequently bypassed in the past when a code was being rereviewed for PC RVU); review of all ultrasonography codes for practice expense; and complete revision of all film processing practice expense to reflect the now-typical digital environment. These aspects have created substantial additional work for the radiology societies' staff and physician volunteers.

Of course, multiple government policies have led to direct regulatory cuts in imaging reimbursement over the past 10 years; these are familiar to those who have been following radiology economics issues, and will not be reviewed in detail here.

Included are the introduction of Evaluation and Management codes (effectively decreasing reimbursement to all other codes approximately 20%); the Deficit Reduction Act of 1996, decreasing technical reimbursement and instituting a technical MPPR; and increases in the equipment utility rate in the 2010 budget, increased in 2011.

Although charges of intentional bias, inadvertent bias, or some combination have been made by the radiology community regarding the excessively burdensome reviews compared with other specialties,[32] the ASNR CPC has remained committed to participating in the CPT/RUC process to maintain its advocacy presence and a voice for the membership. Although there is naturally an urge to "take our marbles and go home" from these bureaucratic minefields, the actual result could be to leave more of our marbles behind.

SUMMARY

The RBRVS has defined the professional reimbursement strategies of CMS, and secondarily of private payors, since its inception in 1992. Radiology groups had a significant influence on the acceptance of this system when it was first introduced, thanks to extraordinary efforts largely through the ACR and its practice leaders, who had been working through various RVS formats before that time. Their success resulted in an entire body of RVU values being accepted in the original Medicare RBRVS, with reaffirmation at the First 5YR. In conjunction with that groundbreaking work, interaction with administrators, payors, legislators, and other stakeholders led to practice models that are still prevalent today: radiology groups independent from hospitals they contract with; component coding structures; and positions of respect attributable to their society advocacy on local and national levels.

Dr Arliss Pollock was a visionary leader of the ASNR, driving the Society and membership to become involved in the AMA House of Delegates, the CPT Panel, and the RUC, while insisting that guidelines, standards, and accreditation programs provide the foundation for procedural recognition and, thereby, reimbursement. ASNR has since been recognized in these forums as a leading society within the radiology and neuroscience communities for its activism.

In recent years many in CMS, MedPAC, Washington, and elsewhere have felt compelled to act on rising health care costs and physician reimbursement distribution, and radiology has become a frequent target of multiple initiatives. The efforts of physician volunteers and staff members from the ASNR, ACR, and SIR, among others, continue to uphold the proud traditions of Arliss Pollock, James Moorefield, and many other radiology leaders who have played critical but rarely heralded roles in the payment policy arena.

ACKNOWLEDGMENTS

I am indebted to ASNR CPC staff Michael Morrow for research work. Additional thanks to ASNR CEO James Gantenberg and ASNR staff Bonnie Mack. The following physicians provided insights and remembrances: David Seidenwurm, MD; Robert M. Barr, MD; Patrick A. Turski, MD; James M. Moorefield, MD; Eric J. Russell, MD; Blake A Johnson, MD; James Borgstede, MD; Bibb Allen, MD; Suresh K. Mukherji, MD. Many thanks for their time and effort.

REFERENCES

1. Moorefield JM, MacEwan DW, Sunshine JH. The radiology relative value scale: its development and implications. Radiology 1993;187:317–26.
2. Russell LB, Manning CL. The effect of prospective payment on Medicare expenditures. N Engl J Med 1989;320:439–44.
3. Hsiao WC, Braun P, Becker E, et al. A national study of resource-based relative value scales for physician services: phase II final report. Boston: Harvard School of Public Health; 1990.
4. Hsiao WC, Braun P, Yntema D, et al. Estimating physicians' work for a resource based relative value scale. N Engl J Med 1988;319:835–41.
5. Lee PR, Ginsburg PB. The trials of Medicare physician payment reform (commentary). JAMA 1991; 266:1562–5. Available at: http://jama.ama-assn.org/content/266/11/1562.full.pdf+html. Accessed June 23, 2012.
6. Oliver TR. Analysis, advice, and congressional leadership: the physician payment review commission and the politics of Medicare. J Health Polit Policy Law 1993;18(1):113–74. DOI:10.1215/03616878-18-1-113.
7. Allen BA. Valuing the professional work of diagnostic radiologic services. J Am Coll Radiol 2007;4(2): 106–14. DOI:10.1016/j.jacr.2006.10.003.
8. Physician payment review commission. Annual report to Congress. Washington, DC: Physician Payment Review Commission; 1989. Available at: http://www.archive.org/details/physicianpayment 00phys. Accessed June 23, 2012.
9. Three of the other RUC seats are physicians elected by the RUC itself on a rotating basis. The other members include the chair, the vice-chair, and the chair of the Practice Expense Subcommittee, who are appointed by the AMA; and liaison representatives from CPT, the American Osteopathic Association, and the Health Care Professionals Advisory Committee.
10. Available at: http://www.ama-assn.org/resources/doc/rbrvs/ruc-update-booklet.pdf. Accessed January 29, 2012.
11. Huckman MS. Dinner at Keen's: the founding of the American Society of Neuroradiology. AJNR Am J Neuroradiol 2001;22:1803–5.
12. Constitution of the American Society of Neuroradiology. Available online at: http://asnr.org/news/ASNR_Constitution.pdf. Accessed January 2, 2012.
13. Mani RL, Eisenberg RL. Complications of catheter cerebral arteriography: analysis of 5,000 procedures. I. Criteria and incidence. AJR Am J Roentgenol 1978; 131(5):861–5.
14. Mani RL, Eisenberg RL. Complications of catheter cerebral arteriography: analysis of 5,000 procedures. II. Relation of complication rates to clinical and arteriographic diagnoses. AJR Am J Roentgenol 1978; 131(5):867–9.
15. Mani RL, Eisenberg RL. Assessment of arteries injected, contrast medium used, duration of procedure, and age of patient. AJR Am J Roentgenol 1978;131(5):871–4.
16. Proceedings of the Annual Meeting of the American Society of Neuroradiology, 2001.
17. Available at: http://www.themonitor.net/Archive/10-25-07/obits.htm. Accessed June 23, 2012.
18. Pollack JA, Turski PA. Representation of the ASNR in the AMA house of delegates at risk. AJNR Am J Neuroradiol 2006;27:239–40.
19. Dillon WP. 2002 presidential address. AJNR Am J Neuroradiol 2002;23(8):1433–5. Available at: http://www.ajnr.org/content/23/8/1433.short. Accessed June 23, 2012.
20. Available at: http://www.ama-assn.org/ama/pub/physician-resources/solutions-managing-your-practice/coding-billing-insurance/cpt/about-cpt/category-iii-codes.page? Accessed June 23, 2012.
21. Gage JO, Krier-Morrow D. What surgeons should know about the "Five-Year Review". Bull Am Coll Surg 2000;85(11):10–3. Available at: http://www.facs.org/ahp/pubs/whatsurg1100.pdf.
22. Available at: http://www.ama-assn.org/ama/pub/physician-resources/solutions-managing-your-practice/coding-billing-insurance/medicare/the-resource-based-relative-value-scale/five-year-reviews.page? Accessed June 23, 2012.
23. Medicare physician payments: fees could better reflect efficiencies achieved when services are provided together. (GAO-09-647). US Government Accountability Office; 2009. Available at: http://www.gao.gov/new.items/d09647.pdf. Accessed January 31, 2012.
24. Mathews AW. Dividing the Medicare pie pits doctor against doctor. Wall St J 2011. Available online at: http://online.wsj.com/article/SB10001424052702303341 904575576480649488148.html. Accessed January 30, 2012.

25. Available at: replacetheruc.org. Accessed June 23, 2012.

26. Donovan WD. What is the RUC? AJNR Am J Neuro-radiol 2011;32:1583–4. Available at: http://dx.doi.org/10.3174/ajnr.A2767. Accessed June 23, 2012.

27. Available at: http://www.slate.com/articles/news_and_politics/prescriptions/2009/09/the_fix_is_in.html. Accessed June 23, 2012.

28. Levy B. The RUC—providing valuable expertise to the Medicare program for twenty years. Kaiser Health News; 2011. Available at: http://www.kaiserhealthnews.org/Columns/2011/March/032811levy.aspx. Accessed January 31, 2012.

29. Medicare payment policy. 2006. p. 133–50. Available at. www.medpac.gov/documents/Mar06_EntireReport.pdf. Accessed June 23, 2012.

30. Available at: medpac.gov/about.cfm. Accessed January 31, 2012.

31. Silva E. New codes from a new source: the rolling five-year review. J Am Coll Radiol 2010;7(1):10–2. DOI:10.1016/j.jacr.2009.10.003.

32. Silva E. The search for misvalued services: why is radiology a target? J Am Coll Radiol 2012;9(1):7–8. DOI:10.1016/j.jacr.2011.10.004.

33. Silva E. CT abdomen and pelvis: a case study in devaluation. J Am Coll Radiol 2011;8(5):300–1. DOI:10.1016/j.jacr.2011.02.008.

34. Available at: https://www.cms.gov/PhysicianFeeSched/PFSFRN/itemdetail.asp?filterType=none&;filterByDID=-99&sortByDID=4&sortOrder=descending&itemID=CMS1253669&intNumPerPage=10. Accessed January 2, 2012.

Accountable Care Organizations for Neuroradiologists
Threats and Opportunities

Frank J. Lexa, MD, MBA[a,b,c,*], Jonathan W. Berlin, MD, MBA[d]

KEYWORDS

• Accountable care organizations • Medical service • Neuroradiologists • Health care quality

KEY POINTS

• Accountable care organizations (ACOs) represent a significant shift in how the Federal government would like to both pay physicians and to control quality.
• Although there are many forms that ACOs can take, at their core they are constructed to reduce costs, to share the cost savings, but to maintain quality standards in the process.
• ACOs represent both a threat and an opportunity for neuroradiologists. Those neuroradiologists who are willing to take on leadership roles in ACOs are likely to thrive compared with their colleagues who participate at the margin of an ACO.
• In the longer term, the ACO model will continue to change; therefore, it is critical that neuroradiologists are vigilant in paying attention to this important change in United States health care.

INTRODUCTION

"We can evade reality, but we cannot evade the consequences of evading reality."
—Ayn Rand[1]

As this article goes to press, accountable care organizations (ACOs) were on schedule to be launched across the United States in January of 2012. Legislatively, they were incorporated into the Federal Health Care Reform Act enacted in 2010.[2] Initially, there was a substantial amount of confusion about what forms they would take and how subspecialists, like those in neuroradiology, would or could participate in these new organizations.

Although there is continuing uncertainty about the mechanics and methods of participation, there seems to be a great deal of flexibility in the form that an ACO could take. That creates an opportunity for specialists to take initiative in creating and

leading an ACO. In fact, neuroradiologists should welcome and, when possible, seek out the opportunity to participate in ACOs and other systems that are paying attention to quality measures and in which neuroradiologists can take on larger roles. In particular, this author would welcome greater latitude in deciding when imaging is appropriate and what the best type of test is in a given situation. Neuroradiologists should welcome the opportunity to participate in building institutional structures in which they can have greater influence on the quality of care. The alternative—being marginalized in a system that is devoted to deemphasizing the role of high technology subspecialists—would be sad outcome for the field.

Neuroradiologists are highly trained subspecialists and are capable of expanding the scope of their involvement with institutions and their colleagues. The default pathway would likely lead to reducing their function to being film readers. The former is

[a] Drexel University College of Medicine, 2900 West Queen Lane, Philadelphia, PA 19129, USA; [b] Global Consulting Practicum, The Wharton School, University of Pennsylvania, Vance Hall, 3733 Spruce Street, Philadelphia, PA 19104, USA; [c] Instituto de Empresa, C/ Maria de Molina, 11 28006, Madrid, Spain; [d] Department of Radiology, NorthShore University HealthSystem, 2650 Ridge Avenue, Evanston, IL 60201, USA
* Corresponding author.
E-mail address: frank22@wharton.upenn.edu

Neuroimag Clin N Am 22 (2012) 437–441
doi:10.1016/j.nic.2012.05.008

the more promising path for neuroradiologists and their groups. However, it is necessary to go into these types of relationships with eyes wide open and to understand the pitfalls as well as the promise of ACOs for advanced neurodiagnosis and treatment modalities.

As this article goes to press, there are still many unanswered questions about ACOs, but that should be a stimulus for attention, not an excuse for avoiding the issues. Although there are many coming changes in health reform in the United States that will affect the profession, vigilant attention to new practice models such as ACOs needs to be paramount. Even if ACOs are not a huge success in their first 3-year outing (a good bet) getting started now will allow neuroradiologists to better adapt to the ACO versions 2.0 and 3.0 that will come next (a fairly safe bet). Finally, the core principles of an ACO—the combination of creating incentives to reduce costs, setting and measuring quality metrics, and promoting longitudinal institutional responsibility for patients—are all likely to be central tenets of health care reform in the United States during the coming decades (almost a sure thing, in fact neuroradiologists should probably bet their careers on it).

A BRIEF HISTORY OF ACOS

ACOs were written into law in H.R. 3590, the Patient Protection and Affordable Care Act (PPACA), in 2010. The initial design by the federal government was significantly built on and influenced by the results of the Center for Medicare and Medicaid Services (CMS) Physician Group Practice Demonstration.[3] In that 5-year demonstration, CMS created a shared savings model with medical groups that allowed the groups to receive payments of up to 80% of the savings generated. The groups were required to adhere to 32 quality measures that were phased in during the 5-year horizon. Costs were tracked for both Medicare Parts A and B spending. Savings were calculated based on growth in costs compared with a base year in the demonstration groups compared with growth in patients in the same local market area who did not receive services from the demonstration groups. The quality metrics included those related to diabetes mellitus, congestive heart failure, coronary artery disease, hypertension, and cancer (breast and colorectal) screening.

Ten groups (Box 1) participated in the demonstration and included approximately 5000 physicians and 220,000 Medicare beneficiaries. There were payments for four performance years. Payments occurred 16 times out of the potential 40 payouts (4 years × 10 participating

---

> **Box 1**
> **Medicare Physician Group Practice Demonstration: participating entities**
>
> Billings Clinic, Billings, Montana
>
> Dartmouth-Hitchcock Clinic, Bedford, New Hampshire
>
> The Everett Clinic, Everett, Washington
>
> Forsyth Medical Group, Winston-Salem, North Carolina
>
> Geisinger Health System, Danville, Pennsylvania
>
> Marshfield Clinic, Marshfield, Wisconsin
>
> Middlesex Health System, Middletown, Connecticut
>
> Park Nicollet Health Services, St. Louis Park, Minnesota
>
> St. John's Health System, Springfield, Missouri
>
> University of Michigan Faculty Group Practice, Ann Arbor, Michigan[3]

---

groups) for a 40% success rate by a pay period measure.

That payout rate should give many readers pause, especially given the high levels of quality and organization represented in the list in Box 1. This is an impressive list of well-run groups in the United States. Although there are advantages and disadvantages to being big, these are groups with some substantial advantages. Whereas some groups did make a fair amount of money, analyzing this by pay period shows that there is real risk of not making money using a shared savings model (at least in some periods) even for outstanding groups. For a group of more average size, running an ACO will be challenging in some circumstances and will require a high degree of planning, organization, and working capital to succeed.

ACOs in 2012—What We Knew in 2011

In March of 2011, the Federal government followed up on the initial legislation of the prior year and released additional information on ACOs in its proposed rules.[4] These included details on many points, including the proposed sharing of savings. These included several critical points that provide insight into how regulators are envisioning the operation of an ACO. The first points of interest are who can be in an ACO and what an ACO can look like:

1. ACO professionals (ie, physicians and hospitals meeting the statutory definition) in group practice arrangements

2. Networks of individual practices of ACO professionals
3. Partnerships or joint ventures arrangements between hospitals and ACO professionals
4. Hospitals employing ACO professionals
5. Other Medicare providers and suppliers as determined by the Secretary Of Health and Human Services.[5]

The second point of interest is how risk is shared. In the proposal, there are two categories of risk sharing. In the first category, the ACO can share in savings, without downside risk for the first 2 years and then must share risk for losses by the third year. In the second category, the ACO assumes both upside and downside risks for the entire 3-year period. The added incentive for the latter is that the percentage of shared savings is higher in the riskier model, 52.5 versus up to 65 cents of each dollar saved, respectively.[6]

Groups will have the option to opt out of the ACO agreement if they give 60 days notice. It might be expected that groups that choose the lower risk path and generate losses will exercise that option before hitting the third year. One hedge that the government has proposed is that it would hold 25% of savings to protect itself against losses later in the arrangement. The ACO will get that cash only if it successfully completes the 3 years.

The third point of interest is how an ACO is set up. An ACO is a legal entity that must apply to the government for a contract. There is no guarantee that an application will be accepted. As previously discussed, there is an opportunity to terminate the relationship before the 3 years are up.

The fourth point of interest is how this interacts with three key legal issues: Stark Law, anti-kickback statutes, and the Civil Monetary Penalty law or anti-gainsharing. A neuroradiologist who is a group leader will need to pay close attention to this and get legal advice if the decision is to join an ACO.

The fifth point of interest is, all of your costs as well as the cash payments from the government must be considered. If, to comply with the regulations, the information technology (IT) infrastructure must be upgraded or additional full-time employees hired in the back office, those costs have to be factored into whether or not the ACO will be successful for the group. In a financial analysis that was published in April of 2011 in the New England Journal of Medicine, the authors suggested that an ACO would require almost a 20% increase in their operating margin to break even in 3 years.[7] This hurdle rate was due to the large up-front investment that was required and was based on data from the Physician Group Practice Demonstration. Although the rules have changed several times in the interim, the initial rules give a great deal of insight into how regulators would prefer to see ACOs run and perhaps a glimpse into how the rules may evolve in the future. The final rules (as of the time that this article goes to press) will be discussed later, but it is important to have a well thought out plan for the group that includes these insights into what is driving the creation of ACOs and perhaps their evolution.

In October of 2011, a final interim rule was released that clarified many of the above points. As this article goes to press, the government is not accepting further comments, so this seems to be the final form for now. However, this is an evolving story, so stay tuned. Further changes are not only likely, they are almost certain to occur. Key changes and updates included:

1. Providers can be added or subtracted during the contract period, thus providing greater flexibility for groups that have turnover in physicians during the contract cycle.
2. Meaningful use (incorporation of effective implementation of IT measures in health care) is a performance measure rather than a baseline requirement.
3. The number of quality measures required for compliance in health care was reduced to 33 from the initial list of 65.
4. Greater transparency about who is a likely beneficiary and there will be provision of a list to allow reconciliation between the ACO and CMS at end of the year.
5. There is an option to avoid downside risk from the beginning and avoid that risk throughout the contract period. Although the reward will be greater for greater risk, this allows groups that are concerned about narrow margins to avoid a direct loss from their ACO participation.
6. There is greater flexibility in start dates and eligibility.
7. The 25% cash withhold is removed.
8. Patients can receive care both within and outside of the ACO.
9. A tax identification number can only be in one ACO, but a provider number can be in more than one. This should give neuroradiologists the opportunity to participate in more than one ACO in some arrangements. As always, stay up-to-date and consult an attorney before signing a contract.
10. A governing board must include ACO participants and meaningful participation by beneficiaries. If there is an opportunity, someone from the group should seek out a leadership role in the ACO, to participate in decision making.

11. Marketing regulations changed from approval requirements to use of a preapproved boilerplate for marketing materials from the ACO.

In addition to this list, there are several additional points that are worth emphasis. First, pay close attention to quality as plans are made and executed for participation in the plan. The rules include adhering to the 33 measures of quality that must be met to succeed as an ACO, as well as compliance with other governance and marketing regulations. Several of my colleagues (the older neuroradiologists) said, on hearing about ACOs, that they have seen this all before in other types of structures that have been built to try to control costs. My answer is, "Not quite." This model is much more sophisticated compared with some of the health maintenance organization (HMO) models from late in the last century. Although many people involved would disagree, many observers have said that many of these models were often focused more on issues such as saving money or gaining market share than on improving health care quality. In an ACO, the quality goals are not only substantial, they are at the core of the model and will be enforced. If quality care is not provided according to those metrics, there will be no reward.

Another point that should be understood is that, although the patients will be assigned to the ACO, they will have the option to opt out of the program. This will necessitate making sure there are enough patients during the contract life to allow for patients who decide to opt out or who leave for other reasons. It also raises an issue that is not completely resolved as this article goes to press—what happens when a patient moves their care around. For example, consider a snowbird who gets her spring and autumn care in Philadelphia, but who summers in Bar Harbor and winters in Palm Beach (not a bad life if you can get it). Developing a transparent method that fairly allocates health care delivery among her providers and also prevents attempts to shift expensive components of care will be a challenge for CMS.

In closing this section, be reminded that the author has deliberately tried to show, not only the final form of the rules, but how they evolved, so that insight can be gained into how regulators view ACOs and how they may morph during a neuroradiologist's career. It should be clear that this is still very much a work in progress and that there are deeper issues that will also need to be worked out. There are potential antitrust issues in health care collaboration as well as the possibility of creating local monopolies. These are only some of the issues that need to be addressed with smart legal help when deciding to join in an ACO. Finally, watch the contracts carefully as they evolve. Right now, CMS has reserved the right to unilaterally change the terms during the contract life, which is a clear legal concern and could conceivably lead to groups deciding to opt out if the changes prove onerous.

ACOs and the Role of Neuroradiologists

Many neuroradiologists who have contacted me about ACO participation seem to have one of two world views: (1) a neuroradiologist has to be in a large university or integrated practice or (2) be working on a contract for a small group of primary care physicians. Both of those models could be part of the future, but I would encourage you to think of other creative ways to participate in ACOs and similar organizations. The key to success or failure in either of the above discussed models (or anything in between) will be how a neuroradiologist sees his or her role. If one is willing to take on a leadership position in the overall care of patients, one's expertise as a neurospecialist will provide value above and beyond one's role as a strong film reader. One element of success will hinge on how well one is able to bring value in many other ways to the institution and its stakeholders. This article closes with a discussion of the neuroradiologist of the future.

TO BE OR NOT TO BE: WHAT IT WILL TAKE TO SUCCEED IN NEURORADIOLOGY IN 2025

There is a quote, attributed to the genius Niels Bohr, that goes, "Prediction is difficult, especially about the future."[8] That should be a reminder that the future is not fixed and it must be considered what the future may hold and, at a profound level, how neuroradiologists might shape the future. It is beyond the scope of this article to consider all of the future scenarios that might be encountered if we rode a time machine into 2025 and observed future neuroradiologists at work, here are two extremes to consider.

Imagine, for the first case, neuroradiologists continue to let a combination of declining government reimbursement, slowed technology innovation, disruptive technologies, and social changes drive them to margin of the roughly 2.5 trillion dollar behemoth that is United States medicine. To attempt to retain income levels, neuroradiologists try to read more films, read faster, and work longer hours. Consequently, they do less research, have less time to spend with clinical colleagues, and have less time to attend conferences or teach outside of subspecialty training programs.

Eventually, medical student interest in neuroradiology falls and research in imaging devolves away from academic radiology programs. Increasingly, other specialties develop their own niche imaging research and training programs and diagnostic radiology declines as a stand-alone specialty. The remaining on-site radiologists in the United States are confined to peripheral roles in medical institutions doing low-value types of imaging. Much of the rest of imaging is done by bulk contracting through national teleradiology companies that are the main source of jobs for young neuroradiologists. Older neuroradiologists who want to continue to work can do so from home by bidding on-line in electronic auctions to read films on an ad hoc basis.

Much of this is already happening, so this is not an imaginary dystopian future. It is a disturbingly likely outcome for at least a substantial number of neuroradiologists. Consider this quote from William Gibson, "The future has already arrived. It's just not evenly distributed yet."[9]

Now imagine an alternative future in which neuroradiologists design protocols for imaging, consult daily on how to customize imaging, work closely with intensive care neurologists to decide on the impact of imaging on care, and give results directly to a significant percentage of outpatients. Imagine further that neuroradiologists are the leaders on most neuroimaging research projects from the basic science level through translational research and comparative effectiveness research. In this future, much of the unnecessary imaging is reduced and is replaced by high-impact protocols and individually tailored imaging. Neuroradiologists are key leaders in the planning of hospital operations in the face of rapidly changing economic, political, and social realities. The United States becomes a laboratory for developing fast, efficient, and effective treatment of the growing burden of neurologic disease in the highly developed world with neuroradiologists at the cutting edge. Pick the future.

SUMMARY

Concluding points are:

1. ACOs are one manifestation of the profound changes that will change the practice of neuroradiology. Ignoring them can imperil a neuroradiologist's practice and career.
2. The concepts and practical issues with ACOs are in a state of flux. Neuroradiologists need to pay very close attention. There have already been substantial changes in the year-long run up to the launch in 2012. It may not be the change that neurologists hoped for, but there will be much more change.

3. There is no single template (at least at the time that this article goes to press) for an ACO. There are many broad categories for how an ACO might be constructed. This reflects a large degree of flexibility in how the government has chosen to launch this experiment. This gives subspecialists in fields such as neuroradiology an unusual opportunity to consider economic models for how to provide care in novel ways.
4. The shared savings component is only a portion of the model. This is not merely a retread of the old HMO model of health care. There will be substantial requirements for how care can be provided. Quality measures have been identified and will be used to insure that the entity delivers rather than merely cuts care.
5. One theme of health reform during the current federal administration has been to shift financial and political power from specialists to primary care physicians. Neuroradiologists will need to have greater visibility and to do compelling research to show their value in the face of this challenge.

REFERENCES

1. Available at: www.Thinkexist.com. Accessed July 17, 2011.
2. The Patient Protection and Affordable Care Act, Senate and House of Representatives of the United States of America, 111th Congress Sess. 2010. Available at: www.govtrack.us/congress/bills/111/hr3590/text. Accessed June 14, 2012.
3. Centers for Medicare and Medicaid Services. Fact sheet: Medicare Physician Group Practice Demonstration: physicians groups continue to improve quality and generate savings under Medicare physician pay for performance demonstration [Internet]. Baltimore (MD): CMS; 2009. Available at: http://www.cms.hhs.gov/DemoProjectsEvalRpts/downloads/PGP_Fact_Sheet.pdf. Accessed July 18, 2011.
4. Available at: https://www.cms.gov/sharedsavings program/. Accessed July 18, 2011.
5. Available at: https://www.cms.gov/MLNProducts/down loads/ACO_NPRM_Summary_Factsheet_ICN906224.pdf. Accessed July 18, 2011.
6. Available at: https://www.cms.gov/sharedsavings program/Downloads/SSPTranscript.pdf. Accessed July 18, 2011.
7. Haywood TT, Kosel KC. The ACO model—a three-year financial loss? N Engl J Med 2011;364:e27. DOI:10.1056/NEJMp1100950. Available at: www.NEJM.org. Accessed November 14, 2011.
8. Available at: http://www.quotationspage.com/quote/26159.html. Accessed November 21, 2011.
9. Available at: www.goodreads.com/author/quotes/9226.William_Gibson. Accessed December 12, 2011.

Certificate of Need

Indu Rekha Meesa, MD, MS[a,b,c,d,e],*,
Robert A. Meeker, MA, MS[c], Suresh K. Mukherji, MD[e]

KEYWORDS

- Certificate of need programs • Health care regulation • Health care legislation • Health care reform

KEY POINTS

- Certificate of Need (CON) is a method of regulating specific health care services at the state level.
- The covered clinical services vary among the individual states.
- CON can assist in reducing health care costs and maintaining quality of patient care if properly administered.

INTRODUCTION

Certificate of Need (CON) programs represent a patchwork of state regulatory programs across the United States that regulate the availability of selected health care services. Thirty-six states maintain laws designed to ensure access to health care services, maintain or improve quality, and control capital expenditures on health care services and facilities by limiting unnecessary health facility construction and checking the acquisition of major medical equipment. This article discusses the history of CON and explores controversies surrounding the current state of CON regulations.

CON legislation originally was introduced by the government in an attempt to solve the cost increase and oversupply problems.[1] This legislation required potential acquirers of medical facilities or technology above a certain monetary value to demonstrate the clinical need for acquiring this capability and qualifications for responsibility of ownership.[2]

CON laws primarily focused on hospitals and nursing homes to halt needless duplication of services and excess capacity. CON regulations were seen as a way to control the "medical arms race" by having organizations demonstrate need for a facility, service, or equipment before investing in them. The term medical arms race implies competition by service expansion and proliferation of new technology. In the 1980s some states expanded their CON regulations to control the proliferation of ambulatory care services as well. Other secondary objectives of CON were to promote access and quality.[3]

Issues surrounding overuse of imaging due to the expansion of availability of imaging centers demonstrate the concept of moral hazard, illustrating supply-driven demand. Moral hazard arises when individuals engage in behaviors under conditions such that their privately taken actions affect the probability distribution of the outcome. By having more scanners in a geographic area, the probability that more studies will be ordered and performed (by virtue of easy access/availability) is increased.

HISTORY OF CON LEGISLATION

In the mid twentieth century, the nation's aging medical infrastructure and workforce were poorly prepared to adequately serve the needs of soldiers

Dr Meesa is now with the University of Michigan Health System, Ann Arbor, Michigan.
[a] Grand Rapids Medical Education Partners, 1000 Monroe Avenue Northwest, Grand Rapids, MI 49503, USA;
[b] Michigan State University, 15 Michigan Street NE, Grand Rapids, MI 49503, USA; [c] Spectrum Health Hospitals, 100 Michigan Street NE, Grand Rapids, MI 49503, USA; [d] Saint Mary's Health Care, 200 Jefferson Avenue SE, Grand Rapids, MI 49503, USA; [e] University of Michigan Health System, 1500 East Medical Center Drive, Ann Arbor, MI 48109, USA
* Corresponding author. University of Michigan Health System, 1500 East Medical Center Drive, Ann Arbor, MI 48109.
E-mail address: rmmeesa@gmail.com

Neuroimag Clin N Am 22 (2012) 443–450
http://dx.doi.org/10.1016/j.nic.2012.05.011
1052-5149/12/$ – see front matter © 2012 Elsevier Inc. All rights reserved

neuroimaging.theclinics.com

returning from World War II and the subsequent increase in the nation's population.[1] There was an insufficient number of hospitals built during the Great Depression, resulting in inadequate medical care for returning soldiers. Congress responded to the situation by passing 2 laws: The Hill-Burton Act of 1946 and the Health Professions Act of 1963. The Hill-Burton Act was passed with the goal of improving medical supply with focus on facility capacity. This act encouraged community planning and hospital construction using Federal subsidies. The Health Profession Act of 1963 focused on the medical workforce. The federal government also expanded access to health care through the Kerr-Mills Act of 1960 for welfare recipients and the 1965 Social Security Act for the elderly and the poor.[4]

Health care spending was rising significantly by the late 1960s. Health care spending had grown at an annual rate of 3.7% in the 1940s and 1950s, but in the 1960s rose at a rate of 5.8%.[1] As a result, the health care expenditures per capita more than tripled between 1940 and 1970.[5] In particular, hospital expenditures more than tripled, to $27.6 billion in a little more than the 10 years from 1960 to 1970.[6]

Three main factors contributed to the rising costs of health care: (1) the implementation of Medicare, (2) the widespread adoption of a traditional fee-for-service (FFS) payment system, and (3) the diffusion of new medical technology. The Medicare health insurance program had a great impact on increasing costs of health care. The Social Security Act signed into law by President Lyndon Johnson on July 30, 1965, established the Medicare and Medicaid health insurance programs. The Medicare program provided health insurance for the elderly and the Medicaid program insured the poor. Through Medicare, currently one of the largest health insurance programs in the world, most elderly patients had nearly full-coverage insurance.[7] As a result, the patients generally ignored the price of the services when choosing a facility. With these plans, patients selected the hospitals based on hospital reputation and their perception of the quality of care provided. In turn, this led hospitals to adopt the latest technology and expand offerings to attract more patients.[3]

The FFS system also contributed to the rising costs of health care. Under FFS, hospitals were reimbursed by insurers for all expenses incurred, regardless of the cost, necessity of the service, or quality of the facility.[1] Under FFS, medical services often expanded beyond their actual need.

The technological change that took place during this period is also another primary cause of rapid increase in health expenditure.[8–10] One of the single most expensive and rapidly diffused medical technologies of that time period was computed tomography (CT) scanning in the mid 1970s.[11] The CT scanner, developed in England by EMI, rapidly changed the diagnostic process for many conditions. Because of its diagnostic capabilities, the CT scanner became rapidly embraced by both patients and clinicians. Sophisticated medical technology is expensive: the unit costs exceed US$1 million.[2] These factors, among others, led to the establishment of CON legislature.

Several steps preceded the common establishment of CON programs by the US states. In an effort to halt rising costs of health care, the federal government and the states decided to implement a health care regulation model originally initiated in Rochester, New York. The Rochester Patient Care Planning Council, composed of insurers, patients, and providers, evaluated the community's hospital needs and determined what services were needed and not needed.[12]

The Comprehensive Health Planning and Services Act signed by President Johnson in 1966 authorized the states to establish planning processes that would rationally allocate federally granted health-related funding.[4] New York established mandatory CON processes in 1966, followed by Maryland, Rhode Island, and District of Columbia.[12] About half of the states had adopted CON laws by 1974.[13] The National Health Planning and Resources Development Act (NHPRDA) of 1974 required the remaining states to establish CON programs[1] that would review and grant approvals to any facility or equipment projects that would expand health care services by any provider.[14]

Only a few years after the CON programs were federally mandated, they came under increasingly severe criticism and, ultimately, were abandoned prematurely by the federal government. During President Ronald Reagan's first term (1981–1985), CON was dismissed by policy makers as an unjustified federal imposition on states and a barrier to competitive dynamics. Congress let the NHPRDA expire in 1986, and federal funding of state CON programs ended the following year.[15,16] Within 2 years, 10 states eliminated their CON programs.[12] In the 1990s and early 2000s, 5 additional states repealed their CON laws in full.[17] While most states have chosen to keep CON, nearly all of them have modified their CON programs to exempt some medical services.[1]

CON AND IMAGING SERVICES

Imaging services are covered by CON laws in most states. Commonly covered imaging services are magnetic resonance (MR) imaging, CT scanning, and positron emission tomography (PET) scanning. However, in some states (eg, Vermont, Maine, District of Columbia, and Hawaii), the basic diagnostic service of ultrasonography requires CON review. The covered services by individual states' CON programs in 2010 are listed in the 2011 American Health Planning Association (AHPA) Directory (available on their Web site, http://www.ahpanet.org). CT, MR imaging, and PET coverage for the individual states are provided by the AHPA 2011 Map Book Certificate of Need coverage (**Figs. 1–4**).

CON regulation of imaging services is controversial. Opponents of CON believe that restricting the development of new imaging services is anticompetitive and impedes patients' access to necessary diagnostic services. In many non-CON states, imaging services are readily available to patients, with little or no waiting time. In CON states where availability of imaging services is restricted, patients may need to schedule their examinations several days in advance and/or during inconvenient hours. Other arguments from the opponents of CON are that CON imposes unnecessary government regulation and that it inhibits the entrepreneurial "spirit."

On the other hand, CON proponents point out that MR imaging, CT, and PET units are costly pieces of equipment and that restricting their numbers ensures optimum use of existing units. Furthermore, many believe that health care facilities generate their own demand, which can be particularly true of diagnostic services such as imaging. In addition, historically imaging services have been a source of positive financial margin for health care providers. Community hospitals, which provide the full spectrum of health care services, often use the margin from imaging services to offset financial losses resulting from other community services, such as 24-hour emergency care and pediatric departments. CON regulations protect community hospitals from independent imaging providers cherry-picking the patients with good insurance coverage, while allowing patients with insufficient or no insurance to go to the community hospitals for diagnostic imaging.

Furthermore, the proponents of CON would say that CON not only limits use and lowers health care costs, as already discussed, it can also discourage nonradiologists from performing complex imaging studies.

CON CONTROVERSIES
Proponents

Although the federal law requiring states to have CON regulations expired in 1986, many states retained CON regulations. Policy makers in many states have been reluctant to completely drop CON laws because of concern that with removal, there might be a surge in health care spending, including both capital expenditures and operating expenses. In fact this is what happened in

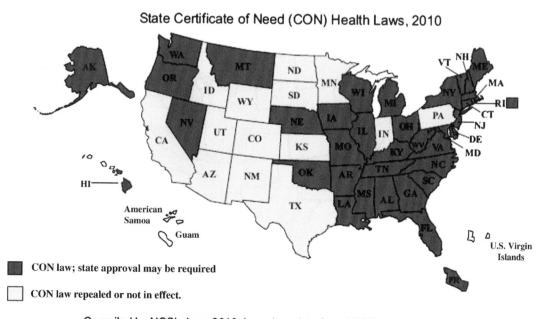

State Certificate of Need (CON) Health Laws, 2010

■ CON law; state approval may be required

□ CON law repealed or not in effect.

Compiled by NCSL June 2010; based on data from AHPA

Fig. 1. Certificate of Need coverage: health laws in the United States, 2010. (*From* American Health Planning Association. Map book: Certificate of Need planning. AHPA; 2011; with permission.)

Certificate of Need: Services Covered
CT Services/Scanners, 2010

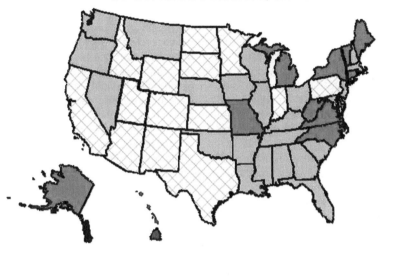

CON Required   No CON Required   No CON Program (14)

Fig. 2. Certificate of Need coverage for computed tomography services. *(From* American Health Planning Association. Map book: Certificate of Need planning. AHPA; 2011; with permission.)

Ohio, which dropped CON requirements for all services except nursing homes in 1998. Ohio experienced an explosion of new ambulatory surgery centers and imaging centers immediately after the CON requirements for these services were eliminated. After removing most CON coverage in Ohio, the state has seen construction of 150 additional surgery centers

Certificate of Need: Services Covered
MRI Services/Scanners, 2010

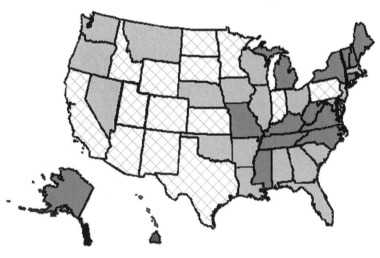

CON Required   No CON Required   No CON Program (14)

Fig. 3. Certificate of Need coverage for magnetic resonance imaging services. *(From* American Health Planning Association. Map book: Certificate of Need planning. AHPA; 2011; with permission.)

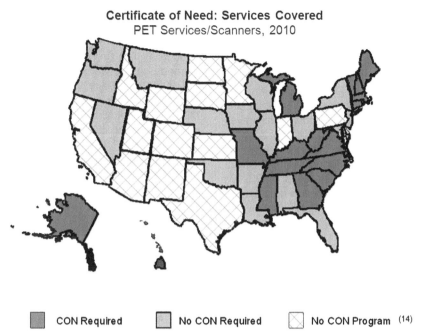

Certificate of Need: Services Covered
PET Services/Scanners, 2010

CON Required   No CON Required   No CON Program (14)

Fig. 4. Certificate of Need coverage for positron emission tomography services. (*From* American Health Planning Association. Map book: Certificate of Need planning. AHPA; 2011; with permission.)

and 300 additional diagnostic imaging centers. These new facilities are often physician owned. After seeing this expansion of ambulatory surgery centers, free-standing dialysis centers, and radiation therapy centers, Ohio proposed reinstating CON law to protect community hospitals.[18] As already discussed, these services tend to be aimed at high profit for hospitals and are badly needed to offset money-draining operations.

According to its proponents the conceptual purposes of CON include that it: functions as a plan implementation tool; supports community-based health services and health facility planning; supports community-oriented planning by health service programs, facilities, and systems; provides analytical discipline and goal orientation in health service and facility planning at all levels; addresses the "excess supply generating excess demand" phenomenon; and limits unnecessary capital outlays.[12]

CON typically focuses on access and quality more than cost. CON regulations seek to improve economic and social access by requiring providers to accept patients regardless of payment source and assure equitable distribution of health facilities. CON elevates quality by promoting best practices and high standards and by establishing minimum volume requirements. Finally, CON promotes fiscal responsibility by requiring providers to use sound economic and planning principles.

CON proponents point to recent studies that demonstrate the success of CON. Faced with rising health care costs and the possibility of weakening or eliminating Michigan's CON program, each of the 3 American automakers undertook separate systematic analyses of their health care costs in states where they have large numbers of employees and insured dependents. DaimlerChrysler Corporation showed that their employees in the non-CON regulated states of Wisconsin and Indiana experienced health care costs almost twice as high as those in the CON states of Delaware, Michigan, and New York. General Motors (GM) analyzed health care use and expense data among its employees and dependents in Indiana, Michigan, New York, and Ohio, 4 states where it has large numbers of insured employees, for the period 1996 to 2001. Comparisons show that GM spent nearly a third less in CON states (New York, Michigan) for health care expenses per employee than in non-CON states (Indiana, Ohio). The study by Ford Motor Company included Kentucky, Michigan, and Missouri (CON states), and Indiana and Ohio (non-CON states). In certain respects, the Ford study is broader than the GM study in that it distinguishes inpatient and outpatient hospital costs, as well as service-specific costs for MR imaging and coronary artery bypass graft surgery. When comparing inpatient and outpatient costs, Ford found that health care costs in

CON states were about 20% lower than in non-CON states.[12]

Opponents

There are several reasons why some states might have chosen to abandon CON laws. During the same time that the desirability of CON was being debated, 2 other types of regulation were developed in an attempt to hold down the costs of health care: The Medicare's Prospective Payment System (PPS) in the 1980s and the Health Maintenance Organization (HMO) Act of 1973. By paying a specified amount for each hospital admission, PPS eliminated hospitals' incentive to inflate costs. In addition to Medicare, more than 30 states adopted rate-setting legislation in the 1980s, which set ceilings on prices that hospitals could charge for certain services.[1] The states followed the lead of the Nixon and Carter administrations, both of which had advocated for increased expenditure controls.[13] The HMO Act of 1973 removed state barriers to managed care. As a result, there was substantial growth of HMOs through the 1980s and managed care in the 1990s.[19] Managed care pressured hospitals to lower costs by negotiating discounted rates. The demand for inpatient hospital care decreased appreciably as a result of growth in managed care planning, as well as implementation of PPS.[3] The lawmakers might have believed that these two regulations (PPS and HMO) along with market pressures would adequately control health care supply and costs without CON regulations.[1] Another big reason could be related to the large amount of empirical evidence accumulated by the early 1980s indicating that CON regulations were ineffective in cost containment.[3]

CURRENT STATUS OF CON

CON laws remain in effect in 36 states and the District of Columbia.

A recent study conducted by the National Institute for Health Care Reform (HCR) compared the CON programs in 6 states: Connecticut, Georgia, Illinois, Michigan, South Carolina, and Washington. Based on telephone interviews with health care stakeholders in each state, the researchers attempted to assess the effectiveness of the CON programs in these 6 states.[20]

In 5 of the 6 states studied, the CON approval process is perceived to be highly subjective. The process is often influenced heavily by political relationships such as provider's clout, organizational size, or overall wealth and resources, rather than policy objectives. The state of Michigan is an exception to this finding.

Michigan is the only state in the study with a formal advisory role for industry stakeholders, employers, consumers, and other interested parties through a CON Commission of 11 members, appointed by the governor. By law, the members of the CON Commission include the following representation: MD representative, DO representative, MD or DO medical school, hospital representative (n = 2), nursing home, nurse, self-insured purchaser, non–self-insured purchaser, labor union, and nonprofit health care organization. The role of the Commission is to establish the rules (called "standards") by which individual CON applications are evaluated.

The Michigan CON Commission relies on issue-specific standards advisory committees (SACs) to recommend changes to the standards for specific CON-covered services (eg, cardiac catheterization, MR imaging, surgical services, and so forth). Membership on the SACs is determined using an open nomination process. By law the composition of a SAC must include a two-thirds majority of subject-matter experts, and representatives of health care provider organizations, health care consumer organizations, health care purchasers, and health care payers. All meetings of the SACs and the Commission are open meetings. Considering recommendations from the SACs and after opportunity for public input, the CON Commission sends proposed CON Review Standards to the State Legislature and the Governor. Either branch of state government can veto the proposed standards. After the specified review period, the new CON Review Standards have the force of law.

The CON Commission does not participate in the review of individual CON applications. Rather, project analysts with the Michigan Department of Community Health evaluate CON applications for compliance with the standards established by the CON Commission. This distribution of responsibility tends to promote greater objectivity and transparency: The appointed commission is responsible for setting CON review standards, and the state Department of Community Health is responsible for the actual review of CON applications.

An overview of the CON application process in the state of Michigan is available at http://www.michigan.gov/mdch/0,4612,7-132-2945_5106-120981–,00.html. An applicant must file a Letter of Intent (LOI) with the Michigan Department of Community Health and a regional review agency, if present. Based on the LOI, the Department will notify the applicant of the required application forms for the proposed project. The corresponding CON application can be submitted online through the Department's CON e-Serve system or by paper to the Lansing Office. Online submission is encouraged to help expedite the application process.

Applications fall into 3 categories: Nonsubstantive, Substantive, and Comparative Review. Nonsubstantive and Substantive applications can be submitted online. Comparative review projects are paper applications. Nonsubstantive reviews involve projects not requiring a full review. Examples include equipment replacements and acquisitions of existing facilities. Substantive reviews involve projects that require a full review on an individual basis, such as a new MR imaging unit or additional units. Comparative reviews involve situations whereby 2 or more applicants are competing for project types for which need is limited.

An applicant must file an application within one of the LOIs as instructed in the Department's notification letter with the required forms and applicable application fee. Within 15 days of receipt of an application, the department reviews it for completeness and requests any additional information as necessary. The applicant has 15 days to submit the requested information.

Once the application is complete, a proposed decision is issued within deadlines for each review type: Nonsubstantive, 45 days; Substantive, 120 days; and Comparative, 150 days. The application is forwarded to the assigned reviewers for an in-depth review of the proposed project. Within the time period the assigned reviewer will prepare a report documenting the analysis and findings of compliance with statutory review criteria and applicable review standards. The reviewer will make a recommendation for approval or disapproval. If the decision is an approval, a final decision is issued by the Department Director within 5 days. If the proposed decision is disapproved, the applicant has 15 days to request a hearing. The hearing must begin within 90 days. Then a final decision is issued by the Department Director following the hearing. If a hearing is not requested, a final decision is issued by the Department Director. There are also opportunities for public input. Any public input received for a particular application will be made part of that application and may be used by the department in its decision. CON application fees are based on total project costs. The fee for projects less than or equal to $500, 000 is $1500; between $500,000 and $4,000,000 is $5500; and equal to or more than $4,000,000 is $8500.

The findings of the HCR study highlight substantial differences among CON programs across the states. In contrast to Michigan, the Illinois Health Facilities and Services Review Board (HFSRB) issues binding decisions on all CON applications filed in the state. Recently wracked by scandal alleging improprieties by Board members, the HFSRB was reformed by 2007 legislation requiring transparency and accountability in all their deliberations.[21]

Even though the CON requirements are not perfect, many respondents believe that CON programs should remain and could be strengthened by moving away from the political influences and focusing on planning policy based on solid data. The CON process can be strengthened with solid state health planning and by improving the process of evaluation and enforcement of CON requirements.[20] CON might be a way to help plan for the evolving dynamics of the local health care market required by health reform coverage expansions and payment reforms.

SUMMARY

CON programs have been maintained in a majority of states, despite substantial changes in the health care arena over the last 40 years. Opinions about the effectiveness of CON vary widely, from concerns about undue government interference in the health care market, on the one hand, to belief that CON programs help to rationalize the health care system and restrain health care cost increases, on the other. Although circumstantial, recent evidence provided by American automobile manufacturers supports the latter opinion. However, until there is proof that implementation of the recent federal health care reform legislation results in lower health care costs, it is unlikely that there will be further erosion in the nation's diverse patchwork of state CON programs, as an antiquated but still moderately effective vanguard against runaway health care costs.

REFERENCES

1. Janelle S. Certificate of Need laws: analysis and recommendations for the commission on rationalizing New Jersey's health care resources, 2007. Available at: http://www.nj.gov/health/rhc/documents/con_laws.pdf. Accessed June 20, 2012.
2. James EA, Perry S, Warner SE, et al. The diffusion of medical technology: free enterprise and regulatory models in the USA. J Med Ethics 1991;17:150–5.
3. Conover CJ, Sloan FA. Does removing certificate-of need regulation lead to a surge in health care spending? J Health Polit Policy Law 1998;23(3): 455–87.
4. Moran DW. Whence and whither health insurance? a revisionist history. Health Aff 2005;24(6):1415–25.

5. Newhouse JP. Economists, policy entrepreneurs, and health care reform. Health Aff 1995;14(1):182–98.

6. Health, United States, 2005. Hyattsville (MD): National Center for Health Statistics. Available at: http://www.cdc.gov/nchs/data/hus/hus05.pdf (2007). Accessed June 20, 2012.

7. Finkelstein A. The aggregate effects of health insurance: evidence from the introduction of Medicare. Q J Econ 2007;122(1):1–37.

8. Newhouse JP. Medicare care costs: how much welfare loss? J Econ Perspect 1992;6:3–21.

9. Fuchs VR. Economics, values, and health care reform. Presidential address of the American Economic Association. Am Econ Rev 1996;86:1–24.

10. Cutler D. Your money or your life: strong medicine for America's health care system. New York: Oxford University Press; 2003.

11. Coulam CM, Erickson JJ, Rollo FD, et al, editors. The physical basis of medical imaging. New York: Appleton-Century-Crofts; 1981.

12. Piper TM. Certificate of need: protecting consumers' interests. Presentation on behalf of the American Health Planning Association to the Federal Trade Commission—Department of Justice Hearing on Health Care competition, quality, and consumer protection: market entry, at the Federal Trade Commission Conference Center (Washington, DC), June 10, 2003.

13. Brown LD. Political evolution of federal health care regulation. Health Aff 1992;11(4):17–37.

14. Choudhry S, Choudhry NK, Brennan TA. Specialty versus community hospitals: what role for the law? Health Aff 2005;(Suppl Web Exclusives):W5361–72.

15. Wiener JM, Stevenson DG, Goldenson SM, et al. Controlling the supply of long-term care providers at the state level. Washington, DC: Urban Institute; 1998.

16. Ho V. Certificate of need, volume, and percutaneous transluminal coronary angioplasty outcomes. Am Heart J 2004;147(3):442–8.

17. American Health Planning Association. National directory; state Certificate of Need programs; Health planning agencies; 2006. Available at: http://www.ahpanet.org/files/ahpa%202006%20directory%20brochure.pdf. Accessed June 20, 2012.

18. Cheryl J. States rethinking need for certificate-of-need laws as fiscal health of hospitals wanes. AMA: 2002. Available at: http://www.ama-assn.org/amednews/2002/07/29/bisb0729.htm. Accessed June 20, 2012.

19. Federal Trade Commission and U.S. Department of Justice. Improving health care: a dose of competition. July 2004. Available at: http://www.ftc.gov/reports/healthcare/040723healthcarerpt.pdf (2007). Accessed June 20, 2012.

20. Yee T, Stark L, Bond A, et al. Health Care Certificate-of-Need Laws: Policy or Politis? National Institute for Health Care Reform, 2011. Available at: http://www.nihcr.org/CON_Laws.html. Accessed June 20, 2012.

21. Dobson AI, Welch WP, Bender D, et al. An evaluation of Illinois' Certificate of Need program. The LEWIN Group. 2007. Available at: http://www.ilga.gov/commission/cgfa2006/Upload/LewinGroupEval CertOfNeed.pdf. Accessed June 20, 2012.

Performance Measures, Efficiency, Productivity

Govind Mukundan, MD, David Seidenwurm, MD*

KEYWORDS

• Performance measurement • Productivity • Efficiency • Structural performance guidelines

KEY POINTS

- Physician performance can be measured objectively.
- There is a Government mandate to promote quality and efficient delivery of health care to help contain costs and cut waste. Physician performance is a key part of this effort.
- Objective criteria for physician performance have an influence on payment.
- Performance standards for neuroradiology have been developed.
- Outcome, process, structure, and satisfaction are domains of performance measurement.
- It is important to account for bias as well as adverse and unintended consequences.
- Health care can be improved by application of objective standards.
- Performance measures, when applied successfully, can objectively validate the trust of the public and payers in the care delivered by physicians and neuroradiology as a whole.

It is the purpose of this order to ensure that health care programs administered or sponsored by the Federal Government promote quality and efficient delivery of health care through the use of health information technology, transparency regarding health care quality and price, and better incentives for program beneficiaries, enrollees, and providers.

—Executive Order of the President, August 26, 2006.

THE PROBLEM

It has long been a fundamental principle of management that you can only manage what you can measure. This dictum is now finding application in the arena of physician and health system payment reform. The issue is no longer whether radiologists' performance will be measured; that is a given. The questions that remain are how and by whom. Another question is whether good performance will be rewarded or bad performance

punished, and what will be the nature of the bonus or malus. Just as consumers of other products demand objective measures of quality, so consumers and their surrogates are demanding that the health care system deliver demonstrable quality. None of us would buy a car without consulting some objective authority regarding the performance parameters we value. Reliability, safety, and economy are considered basic criteria for these judgments, and we certainly take subjective factors such as style, handling, and performance characteristics into account. Consumers of health care, via their surrogates such as insurance companies, and payers such as employers and taxpayers, through their representatives in government, demand nothing less of us.

The public recognizes both the importance and the high cost of imaging. Most concerns revolve around cost and quality, or as President George W. Bush succinctly put it, "transparency regarding health care quality and price." Much of this concern is fueled by the startling growth of health care costs in the United States over time, from around 3% of gross domestic product (GDP) in

Neuroradiology, Radiological Associates of Sacramento, 1500 Expo Parkway, Sacramento, CA 95815, USA
* Corresponding author.
E-mail address: SeidenwurmD@radiological.com

Neuroimag Clin N Am 22 (2012) 451–456
doi:10.1016/j.nic.2012.05.009
1052-5149/12/$ – see front matter © 2012 Elsevier Inc. All rights reserved.

neuroimaging.theclinics.com

the 1940s to 17.3% in 2009[1] while the relative cost of other goods and even some services has declined (Fig. 1).[2]

It is also relevant that the United States system, in the aggregate, produces worse results at higher costs than those of other countries. Indeed, the debate on cost control in radiology closely mirrors that of the global health care debate in this country.

Equally compelling is the question of utilization. Radiology especially has become a target of utilization review, given the steep climb in recent years in quantity and costs of expensive imaging tests and procedures.[3] We are asked: are all the tests being performed really necessary? The paradox of increased use without obvious evidence of improved health outcomes has led to calls for payment based on value rather than volume. Measurement of radiologists' performance is a key component of the measurement of value.[4]

THE FRAMEWORK

Pay for performance is defined as any payment scheme that explicitly tries to align the incentives of the provider with that of the patient; this has not always been the case in the past. For example, the Medicare Payment Advisory Commission in 2003 stated "the Medicare payment scheme is largely neutral or negative toward quality... At times providers are paid even more when quality is worse, such as when complications occur as a result of error." In a fee-for-service environment, volume is rewarded while quality is not, except in those circumstances whereby high-quality providers capture a greater market share as a result of their reputation for excellence.

Defining performance and quality, and setting up a feasible scheme for aligning quality with payment, have therefore become a central component in the health care debate, given the growth of health care spending in absolute as well as relative terms as a share of GDP, and the attendant questions regarding use and effectiveness.

Primary assumptions for the theoretical development of performance measures include the following:

1. Medical doctors are human from a management standpoint.
2. As humans, they respond to incentives.
3. Patients and/or their surrogates need information to make choices.
4. Health care, and radiology within this framework, is a rational enterprise.

Rational decision makers will choose the highest quality at the best price. The introduction of management techniques has been shown to increase productivity and reduce cost in other enterprises.[5] Assuming that health care and thus radiology are rational human enterprises, it can be postulated that application of effective management techniques to health care and thus radiology can also improve productivity and reduce cost and waste. Indeed this has been shown to be the case, as pay-for-performance measures, even with small incentives, have been shown to improve quality of care in comparison with control groups.[6,7]

The reference point for performance measurement can also be controversial. Under the standard medical paradigm of care, we try to establish a single threshold for risk versus benefit for an intervention. Once this is reached, the doctor suggests the intervention. In a more patient-centered world, several thresholds may exist. These thresholds would include one under which no intervention would take place, an intermediate zone where undergoing the intervention is left to the patient's discretion, and a third threshold where an intervention is clearly recommended.[8] Such a scenario is important because physicians and patients differ systematically in the perception of risk, especially when domains of disability are not the same. For example, in a study by Guyatt and colleagues,[9] physicians and patients differed widely regarding how many gastrointestinal bleeds they were willing to tolerate to prevent a stroke. Thus, the discretionary range may be quite large, or the thresholds may be set

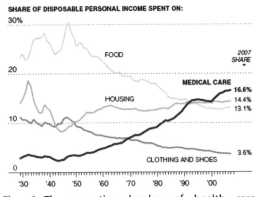

SHARE OF DISPOSABLE PERSONAL INCOME SPENT ON:

Fig. 1. The mounting burden of health care. Spending on health care, which takes up more of consumers' income than housing, food, or clothing, has risen significantly since 2000. As the economy slows and medical costs continue to increase, millions of people may be unable to afford care. (Available at: http://www.nytimes.com/imagepages/2008/05/04/business/20080504_INSURE_GRAPHIC.html. Copyright 2008, the New York Times Company; with permission.)

via social consensus at cutoff points that seem puzzling to technically oriented physicians. Finally, interventions based on principles of evidence-based medicine yield better outcomes at reduced cost than non–evidence-based practices.

Central to pay for performance is performance itself. How do we measure this? How do we rationally develop a methodology to measure and reward performance in radiology?

PROCESS FOR THE DEVELOPMENT OF RADIOLOGY PERFORMANCE MEASURES

Defining performance measures is a complex task. Pitfalls include patient selection bias by providers, that is, some providers may avoid patients with complex and difficult medical problems to prevent scoring lower on performance. In neuroradiology, this might be an interventional neuroradiologist actively selecting patients with fewer comorbidities for procedures and referring those with complex medical problems to another institution to maintain a pristine complication rate, a measure of performance. It must be noted that sometimes this would be beneficial, as those patients with extensive comorbidities may be less likely to benefit in the long term from complex interventions.

A diagnostic neuroradiologist in theory might decline to evaluate or read computed tomography (CT) angiograms of the neck and head in patients with Loeys-Dietz or Ehlers-Danlos syndrome, knowing that the turnaround time (a metric for performance) for a report would be longer, owing to a more complex examination, than for a less complex patient.

This situation can lead to safety-net providers taking on a disproportionate number of these more complicated patients, leading to a performance shift in the health care ecosystem without any real net gain in performance as a whole. Also, to the extent that pay would be tied to performance, those systems whose resources are already strained might be disadvantaged even more.

Other potential problems include "teaching to the test" whereby providers and health care institutions try to follow procedures that are aimed at maximizing performance scores at the expense of true quality of health care. A radiologist might be distracted by the need to report the National Institute of Neurological Disorders and Stroke exclusion criteria to qualify for the PQRS (Physician Quality Reporting System) bonus, and overlook the obstructive hydrocephalus that accounts for the patient's decreased level of consciousness.

The process for the development of radiology performance measures seeks to address the potential impact on quality, gaps in care, existing guidelines, and current literature, taking into account regional variation. The best performance measures are those that are based on multiple-specialty practice guidelines[10] that are themselves grounded in evidence-based medicine, are consensus driven, and are validated in clinical practice.

Best performance measures:

1. Based on multi-specialty guidelines
2. Evidence based
3. Face valid
4. Construct valid
5. Large denominator
6. Multi-stakeholder process
7. Testing validated
8. Severity adjusted
9. Updated systematically

However, these are plagued by constantly evolving advances in published data, conflicts of interest, turf battles, and narrow scope, and can be inadequate for covering complex patient cases. Despite these limitations, dozens of performance measures relevant to radiology are in use around the country, and one or more of them directly or indirectly affect virtually all radiologists (Box 1).

Outcome measures directly measure a health variable, for example, complication rate in interventional neuroradiology or mammography call-back rate. Potential pitfalls include methodology for measurement, adverse patient selection, assignment to specific neuroradiologists, need for risk adjustment, and accounting for potential lag

---

Box 1
Types of performance measures

1. Outcome. Directly measures health variable, for example, death or survival rate, diabetic control, mammography call-back rate, complication, turnaround time

2. Process. Measures adherence to accepted practice patterns, for example, timely work-up of transient ischemic attack (TIA), use of NASCET (North American Symptomatic Carotid Endarterectomy Trial) method, individual CT dose protocols

3. Structural. Evaluates inputs such as personnel or resources, for example, board-certified neuroradiologists, magnetic resonance (MR) imaging accreditation, mammography audit database

4. Satisfaction. Surveys patient opinions, for example, waiting time, comfort, subjective perceptions of overall care quality

time between intervention and effect (time to measurement).

Process measures quantify adherence to accepted practice guidelines, for example, CT radiation dose protocols or the use of the NASCET method for quantification of carotid stenosis. Pitfalls include following the process to the detriment of individual patient care, "cookbook" medicine, or optimizing documentation rather than actual care. This problem can become real rather than theoretical in practices that use electronic medical records or structured report templates.

Structural performance measures inputs such as personnel, equipment such as board certification for radiologists, or American College of Radiology accreditation for MR imaging scanners. Pitfalls include waste when the costs of creating the structure exceed the benefits, or if the prima facie value of an accepted structure of care does not result in improved outcomes. Measures of patient satisfaction or experience of care quantify subjective perceptions of quality and patients' experience. Being subjective, these concepts are difficult to measure and are expectation dependent. For example, a patient who is used to poor care may find average wait times at an outpatient center to be outstanding, whereas another patient who is used to concierge medicine may find an average wait time to be below par. Satisfaction measures may result in radiologists diminishing patients' expectations to exceed them. Like the experience at the car dealer's service department, one might attempt to optimize performance by coaching the patient on survey responses.

Performance measures, because they are necessarily quantitative, require a specific variable to be evaluated. Then one needs to set a threshold for performance. These thresholds can be absolute, for example a complication or miss rate or recall rate below a certain number, or relative, for example a complication rate relative to peers, or improvement based, that is, improvement of a patient score or provider's performance over time. Each of these approaches can have adverse consequences if the level of performance is tied to remuneration or other consequences. For example, below-average performers in resource-deprived institutions might see financing worsen, creating a vicious cycle, or high performers might forgo opportunities to improve if they have reached the maximum potential bonus.

Finally, there has to be an adjustment for the complexity or severity of the types of patients being treated by providers. For example, a neuroradiologist dealing with complex head and neck and central nervous system tumor cases in a tertiary care center is dealing with a very different patient population from that of a neuroradiologist in a community setting seeing largely a mix of lumbar spine imaging evaluations for radiculopathy and brain imaging evaluations for headaches. In general, it is best to create measures that do not require severity adjustment. For example, the studies justifying the use of breast MR imaging in high-risk women had mammography recall rates similar to those prevailing in average-risk women, suggesting that a performance measure for mammography recall does not require severity adjustment. Similarly, patients with TIA and patients with completed strokes need timely evaluation for surgical disease of the brain and the blood vessels within the broadest range of severity. Furthermore, the distribution of case severity is less skewed than many physicians believe. After all, everyone's patients can't be sicker than everyone else's.

PROCESS FOR ENDORSEMENT OF RADIOLOGY MEASURES

Because measurement of radiologist performance is in its infancy, the data on the actual impact of performance measurement is sparse. Consensus-based measures, developed with input from a broad base of stakeholders, are a necessary starting point. These measures require testing and validation in practice, just like any other medical procedure or diagnostic test. Moreover, it is crucial to understand that the metrics for evaluation of performance are similar to those that evaluate the diagnostic tests we perform daily. For this reason, most performance measures are subject to frequent reevaluation and testing for reproducibility and feasibility in practice, validity, and other parameters.

It is useful to study the recommendations of the Institute of Medicine committee directed under the US Congress to study alignment of performance of payers to performance for the Medicare program under the Title XVIII of the Social Security Act (42 U.S.C 1395 et seq.).[11] This committee, made up of individuals from the various stakeholders in the health care arena, recommended a phased approach for the introduction, evaluation, and modification of performance measures to providers. Following evaluation and analysis of the data from these initial trials, larger trials with multiple measures and reward settings can be introduced, thus allowing evaluation of the efficiency and efficacy of each performance measure, and a better understanding of unintended effects, bias, and so forth of each trial.

Development of performance measures in radiology is in many ways analogous to that in other areas of medicine. However, there are also important differences that must be understood. The first is obvious: radiologic end points are primarily based on diagnosis whereas other specialties are treatment driven. For example, for a radiologist, determining a diagnosis of acute appendicitis on a CT of a patient and communicating a report to the referring physician in a timely manner constitutes his or her sole involvement in the episode of that patient's care. Therefore developing a performance measure, for example an accurate diagnosis, is very different than one developed for the surgeon who operates on the patient and whose performance is based on the outcome of the surgery. One could argue that the outcome of the patient, if poor because of the surgery, could have had very little to do with the radiologist, as long as the interpretation was conducted and transmitted appropriately. Thus the performance measure to evaluate the radiologist would have to account for this. Alternatively one might simply evaluate at the level of the system of care or payer, and create a more global incentive for performance improvement.

Another attribute unique to radiology is radiation dose. We potentially do harm when we scan our patients with ionizing radiation or a nuclear medicine isotope. Thus, performance measures based on dose mitigation are very different from those of treatment-driven medicine (**Table 1**).

High-impact areas for performance measures in neuroradiology could include:

1. Stroke
2. Back pain, neck pain
3. Headache
4. Seizure
5. Sinus disease
6. Iodinated and gadolinium contrast dose
7. Radiation dose

Performance measures related to these topics are either in use or under consideration.

The lead in development of clinical performance measures in radiology has been taken under the PQRS, formerly known as PQRI, established under the Tax Relief and Health Care Act of 2006,[12] using the American Medical Association (AMA) convened Physician Consortium for Performance Improvement (Consortium) and the National Committee for Quality Assurance. Although some of these performance measures are designed for individual quality improvement, most of these measures can be appropriate for accountability, assuming that these stand up to methodological, statistical, and postimplementation scrutiny.

In the end, the paradigm shift occurring in radiology and health care as a whole may seem daunting to the radiologist with the clamor for increasing accountability from payers and patients alike. However, it is through powerful tools such as performance measures in radiology and the incentive-based payment systems that accompany them that we, as physicians, can improve our practices and restore the confidence of our patients and society as a whole in what we do and should be doing: treating patients effectively in an optimal manner every time.

Table 1
Performance measures in radiology compared to other medical specialties

Radiology	Other Non–Imaging-Based Specialties
End points largely diagnosis driven	End points largely treatment driven
Radiation dose/MR imaging specific absorption rate	Not usually a consideration with the exception of radiation oncology (analogous to surgical blood loss, undesirable but unavoidable impact of care)
Contrast dose, gadolinium or iodinated contrast	Not usually applicable (analogous to use of opiate pain relief in low back pain, elective, potentially avoidable exposure to complications)

REFERENCES

1. The Centers for Medicare and Medicaid Services. National health expenditure projections 2009-2019. Available at: https://www.cms.gov/NationalHealth ExpendData/downloads/proj2009.pdf. Accessed June 22, 2012.
2. Available at: http://www.nytimes.com/imagepages/ 2008/05/04/business/20080504_INSURE_GRAPHIC. html. Accessed June 22, 2012.
3. Shikles JL. Physicians who invest in imaging centers refer more patients for more costly services. In: United States General Accounting Office. Testimony before the subcommittee on health, committee on ways and means. Washington, DC: U.S. House of Representatives; 1993. Publication GAO/T-HRD-93-14:149–63.
4. Seidenwurm D, Turski P, Barr J, et al. Performance measures in neuroradiology. AJNR Am J Neuroradiol 2007;28:1435–8.
5. Bloom N, Eifert B, Mahajan A, et al. Does management matter? Evidence from India. Cambridge (MA): National Bureau of Economic Research; 2011.

6. Campbell SM, Reeves D, Kontopantelis E, et al. Effects of pay for performance on the quality of primary care in England. N Engl J Med 2009;361: 368–78.

7. Peterson LA, Woodard L, Urech T, et al. Improving patient care: does pay-for-performance improve the quality of health care? Ann Intern Med 2006; 145:265–72.

8. Quanstrum KH, Hayward RA. Lessons from the mammography wars. N Engl J Med 2010;363:1076–9.

9. Guyatt GH, Oxman AD, Vist GE, et al. GRADE: an emerging consensus on rating quality of evidence and strength of recommendations. BMJ 2008;336: 924–6.

10. Seidenwurm DJ, Davis PC. Evidence based imaging of the nervous system. AJNR Am J Neuroradiol 2007;28:798.

11. Institute of Medicine. Rewarding provider performance: aligning incentives in Medicare. 2006. Available at: http://www.iom.edu/Reports/2006/Rewarding-Provider-Performance-Aligning-Incentives-in-Medicare.aspx. Accessed June 22, 2012.

12. Available at: https://www.cms.gov/PQRS/. Accessed June 22, 2012.

National Initiatives for Measuring Quality Performance for the Practicing Neuroradiologist

Nikesh Anumula, MD[a], Pina C. Sanelli, MD, MPH[a,b],*

KEYWORDS

- Physician Quality Reporting System • Quality measures • Incentive payment
- Hospital Outpatient Quality Data Reporting Program • Outpatient imaging efficiency
- Hospital Outpatient Prospective Payment System

KEY POINTS

- The Physician Quality Reporting System is an incentive payment program for eligible physicians who satisfactorily report data on quality measures.
- The Hospital Outpatient Quality Data Reporting Program is a pay-for-quality data reporting program for outpatient hospital services.
- The Hospital Outpatient Prospective Payment System is used by the Centers for Medicare and Medicaid Services to reimburse for hospital outpatient services.

INTRODUCTION

This article provides an overview of national initiatives developed for monitoring and reporting quality performance measures. Included are a review of the Physician Quality Reporting System (PQRS), the Hospital Outpatient Quality Data Reporting Program (HOP QDRP), and the Hospital Outpatient Prospective Payment System (HOPPS), with specific emphasis on how these programs affect radiology practice. These programs are operated by federal agencies to measure and monitor the quality of healthcare practices at the individual physician and hospital levels, and for the implementation and regulation of an effective system of reimbursement. These programs are under the jurisdiction of the Centers for Medicare and Medicaid Services (CMS), previously known

as the Health Care Financing Administration, which is a federal agency within the US Department of Health and Human Services that administers the Medicare program and works in partnership with states to administer Medicaid and the State Children's Health Insurance Program. A practical review of these programs allows radiologists to gain further understanding of the economic and political influences on the daily practice of radiology today. The background and relevant features of each program are presented in this review.

PHYSICIAN QUALITY REPORTING PROGRAM
Overview

This section provides a brief review of the PQRS, highlighting the program's legislative history, eligibility requirements, and incentive payment plan.

a Department of Radiology, Weill Cornell Medical College, New York-Presbyterian Hospital, 525 East 68th Street, Starr Pavilion, New York, NY 10065, USA; b Department of Public Health, Weill Cornell Medical College, New York-Presbyterian Hospital, 402 East 67th Street, New York, NY 10065, USA
* Corresponding author. Department of Radiology, Weill Cornell Medical College, New York-Presbyterian Hospital, 525 East 68th Street, Starr Pavilion 8A, New York, NY 10065.
E-mail address: pcs9001@med.cornell.edu

Neuroimag Clin N Am 22 (2012) 457–466
doi:10.1016/j.nic.2012.04.010
1052-5149/12/$ – see front matter © 2012 Elsevier Inc. All rights reserved.

The PQRS program began in 2007 to provide an incentive payment to eligible physicians who satisfactorily report data on quality measures for covered Physician Fee Schedule (PFS) services furnished to Medicare Part B Fee-for-Service beneficiaries. Specifically, the PQRS measures applicable to the practice of neuroradiology are discussed. Several steps are suggested for individual physicians or group practices to start participation in the program. Resources are also provided for further information on the program requirements and the individual PQRS measures.

History and Background

The PQRS program is a relatively new program but has experienced a gradual process of transition since its inception. In 2006, the Tax Relief and Health Care Act[1] established this program as an initiative to provide a 1.5% incentive payment with a cap for eligible physicians who satisfactorily reported data on quality measures for covered services furnished to Medicare. In 2007 the Medicare, Medicaid, and State Children's Health Insurance Program Extension Act[2] authorized continuation of the PQRS program for 2008 and 2009, which also provided a 1.5% incentive payment in 2008 and removed the cap established by the Tax Relief and Health Care Act. In 2008, the Medicare Improvements for Patients and Providers Act[3] established the PQRS as a permanent federal program. It also increased the incentive payment to 2% of the total allowed charges for PFS-covered professional services in 2008 and 2009.

The Affordable Care Act,[4] signed into law by President Obama in 2010, made several changes to the PQRS program. These changes included a gradual decrease in the incentive payment, requiring that quality measures eventually be met to receive the maximum Medicare payment for services. In 2011, the program decreased the incentive payment to 1% of the total allowed charges for PFS-covered professional services. The incentive will be further decreased to 0.5% in 2012 through 2014 and will eventually become a penalty starting in 2015 if not met. The expected starting penalty is a 1.5% reduction in the total allowed charges for PFS-covered professional services. In 2016, there will be further reduction to 2% in payment for services if the reporting measures are not met.[4]

Quality Performance Measures

The PQRS program consists of more than 200 quality measures for Medicare patients including various aspects of care, such as prevention, chronic and acute care management, procedure-related care, resource use, and care coordination. Fifteen of these quality measures are applicable to diagnostic radiology, interventional radiology, or nuclear medicine as shown in Table 1.

The following three measures are applicable to most neuroradiologists in practice[5]:

1. *Measure 10—Stroke and Stroke Rehabilitation: CT or MR Imaging Reports* refers to the percentage of finalized reports for CT or MR imaging studies within 24 hours of arrival to the hospital for patients aged 18 years and older with either a diagnosis of ischemic stroke or transient ischemic attack or intracranial hemorrhage or at least one documented symptom consistent with ischemic stroke or transient ischemic attack or intracranial hemorrhage that include documentation of the presence or absence of each of the following: (1) hemorrhage, (2) mass lesion, and (3) acute infarction.
2. *Measure 195—Stenosis Measurement in Carotid Imaging Reports* refers to the percentage of final reports for all patients, regardless of age, for carotid imaging studies (including neck MR angiography, neck CT angiography, carotid duplex sonography, and carotid angiography) performed that include direct or indirect reference to measurements of the distal internal carotid artery diameter as the denominator for the stenosis measurement.
3. *Measure 145—Radiology Exposure Time Reported for Procedures Using Fluoroscopy* refers to the percentage of final reports for procedures using fluoroscopy that include documentation of the radiation exposure or exposure time.

Program Requirements

The PQRS is a voluntary incentive program. Submission of quality data codes through claims or a qualified registry indicates the intent to participate. In claims-based individual reporting, each eligible physician must report a minimum of three measures if applicable to his or her practice.[6] There must be 50% compliance in a minimum of three measures to qualify for the incentive payment.[6] However, if an eligible physician has less than three measures applicable to their practice, they are still able to participate in the program reporting on only their applicable measures.[6] If fewer than three measures are reported, CMS may apply a measure-applicability validation process to determine eligibility for the incentive payment.[6]

CMS uses two methods for assessing conformity to the requirements, referred to as "reporting compliance" and "quality compliance."[7] Reporting compliance reflects the percentage of eligible

Table 1
PQRS measures applicable to radiology

Category	Measure No	Title
Stroke and stroke rehabilitation	10	CT or MR imaging reports
Perioperative care	20	Timing of antibiotic prophylaxis, ordering physician
Perioperative care	21	Selection of prophylactic antibiotic, first or second-generation cephalosporin
Perioperative care	22	Discontinuation of prophylactic antibiotics (noncardiac procedures)
Perioperative care	23	Venous thromboembolism prophylaxis (when indicated in all patients)
Prevention of catheter-related bloodstream infections	76	Central venous catheter insertion protocol
Health information technology	124	Adoption/use of electronic health records
Medication reconciliation	130	Documentation of current medications in the medical record
Radiology	145	Exposure time reported for procedures using fluoroscopy
Radiology	146	Inappropriate use of "probably benign" assessment category in mammography screening
Nuclear medicine	147	Correlation with existing imaging studies for all patients undergoing bone scintigraphy
Preventive care and screening	173	Unhealthy alcohol use, screening
Radiology	195	Stenosis measurement in carotid imaging reports
Radiology	225	Reminder system for mammograms
Preventive care and screening	226	Tobacco use: screening and cessation intervention

Data from American College of Radiology. Physician Quality Reporting System updates. Available at: http://www.acr.org/Quality-Safety/Quality-Measurement/Value-Based-Purchasing/PQRS/Resources.

cases that have a PQRS code assigned. The incentive plan is based on obtaining reporting compliance. The physician performance data are published on-line as a list of the eligible professionals who satisfactorily report PQRS measures since 2009. Quality compliance refers to the percentage of reported cases that have completed the quality measure. Currently, quality compliance data are collected and monitored by CMS. Compliance is measured as a ratio: "denominator" refers to all eligible cases for a particular measure in your practice, and "numerator" refers to successful reporting of the measure.

The beginning of this year's cycle is January 1, 2012. However, you can start participating in the program during the mid-year cycle. **Fig. 1** demonstrates five main steps to getting started.[8]

Resources

More information and details can be found at the Centers for Medicare and Medicaid.[9] A brief synopsis of the PQRS program can be found in the *American Journal of Neuroradiology*.[10]

HOSPITAL OUTPATIENT QUALITY DATA REPORTING PROGRAM
Overview

A brief review of HOP QDRP is provided, highlighting the program's legislative history, outpatient imaging efficiency (OIE) measures, and payment plan. Specifically, HOP QDRP measures applicable to imaging practices are discussed. Resources are also provided for further information and details.

History and Background

HOP QDRP is a pay for quality data reporting program implemented by CMS for outpatient hospital services. This program was instituted by the Tax Relief and Health Care Act of 2006 and requires hospitals to submit data on measures regarding the quality of care provided in the outpatient setting. Measures of quality include those related to process, structure, outcome, and efficiency.

The purpose of these outpatient measures is to evaluate the consistency with which a healthcare provider administers the best known available outpatient care for a particular condition. Specifically for radiologists, the goal is to promote high-quality

Step 1: Determine whether you are eligible to participate. A list of professionals who are eligible is provided on the CMS website (www.cms.hhs.gov).

Step 2: Determine which reporting option best fits your practice (claims-based or registry-based reporting of either individual measures or group measures).

Step 3: Determine which PQRS measures are applicable to your practice. Eligible professionals who choose to report individual measures should select at least 3 applicable measures to qualify for the incentive payment. If fewer than 3 measures are reported, CMS may apply the measure-applicability validation (MAV) process to determine eligibility for the incentive payment.

Step 4: Review the following documents: (a) *Physician Quality Reporting System Measure Specifications Manual for Claims and Registry* (http://www.acg.gi.org/members/nataffairs/thisweek/2011PQRSMeasureSpecificationManualfor ClaimsandRegistryReporting.pdf) provides instructions for reporting claims or registry-based measures. A review of the documents for the current year should be performed.
(b) *Physician Quality Reporting System Implementation Guide* (http://www.astro.org/PublicPolicy/PQRIInformation/documents/2011implementationguide.pdf) describes the important reporting principles and rationale for each measure.

Step 5: Proper documentation is needed in your reports to qualify for the measures. Developing templates for standardized reporting may be helpful. Review the operational procedures in your practice to ensure accurate reporting. Education of the staff, billing office, residents, and fellows (if applicable) is important for obtaining compliance.

Fig. 1. Five steps to enroll in the PQRS program. (*Adapted from* Centers for Medicare & Medicaid Services. Physician quality reporting system: how to get started. Available at: http://www.cms.gov/Medicare/Quality-Initiatives-Patient-Assessment-Instruments/PQRS/How_To_Get_Started.html.)

efficient care, reduce unnecessary exposure to contrast materials or radiation, and promote adherence to evidence-based medicine practice guidelines. In addition to providing hospitals with a financial incentive to report their quality of care measure data, the program provides CMS with data to help Medicare beneficiaries make more informed decisions about their health care. Hospital quality of care information gathered through this program is available on the *Hospital Compare* Web site (www.hospitalcompare.hhs.gov).[11]

Quality Performance Measures

Outpatient imaging is an essential component of the healthcare system, providing important tools in the diagnosis, management, and treatment of disease. To date, there have been few efforts to implement national standards and quality control in the delivery of these services, thus precluding the ability to monitor the success or track-record of radiology practices in the United States. In this respect, the establishment of OIE measures can help define measurable indicators, such as appropriate use, excellence in technical performance, timeliness in study reporting, and clinical effectiveness and efficiency to improve the quality of radiology practice at the national level.

Efficiency can be defined as the "absence of waste" in clinical practice. The Institute of Medicine has defined efficiency as avoiding the use of resources that do not provide any benefit to patients and classifies the use of such resources as "waste." The Research and Development

Corporation has defined "clinical waste" as the provision of clinical services for which the cost of the service outweighs the benefit. These OIE measures are classified within six domains as shown in **Table 2**.

CMS is currently using 14 measures in HOP QDRP and each measure must meet the four criteria in **Table 3** to be implemented. Seven of the measures (OP-8–11 and OP-13–15) are OIE measures and are of interest to radiologists. These measures are described in **Table 4**.

Program Requirements

In this program, hospitals that do not successfully meet the administrative data collection, submission, validation, and publication requirements receive a 2% reduction in their annual payment update (APU) under HOPPS.[12] Please refer to the following section for more information on the HOPPS program. HOP QDRP is different from the PQRS program previously described. The PQRS is a voluntary program that offers an incentive payment when the requirements are successfully met. The HOP QDRP is calculated on a per-hospital basis, whereas the PQRS is calculated on a per physician or group practice basis.[12]

Exclusion criteria are used to restrict the scope of the OIE measures to clinical circumstances that are guided by evidence-based guidelines and research evidence. The exclusions applied to each measure serve to standardize the measures across providers, eliminate cases for which there is expected to be little variation, and eliminate cases for which there is little agreement on the correct clinical course. Please refer to the CMS Web site (www.cms.gov) for further details regarding exclusion criteria for each measure.

For public reporting purposes, there must be an adequate number of cases in the measure's denominator. If a hospital outpatient department performs a small number of imaging studies meeting the measure's specifications, the observed value may be an unreliable indicator of a hospital's true performance. Thus, the CMS established minimum case counts for each measure. If a hospital does not meet the minimum case count for public reporting, *Hospital Compare* does not report the data for these imaging measures. The minimum case count requirements are different for each measure and apply specifically to each observed percentage value.[13] For example, if the facility rate for a given measure is 0.1 or 10%, the required precision is ± 6% and the case count needed to obtain that level of precision is 66. If the frequency is 0.5 or 50%, the required precision is 15% and the minimum case count is 31. As the facility rate increases, the degree of precision decreases and consequently the minimum number of denominator cases needed to reach that level of precision decreases. These values are based on obtaining a 90% confidence interval for a given facility rate. A more thorough description of minimum case counts can be found at the following web address: https://www. cms.gov/HospitalQualityInits/Downloads/Hospital OutpatientImagingEfficiencyMinimumCaseCounts. pdf.

Eligibility

Currently, all acute-care hospitals are required to enroll in HOP QDRP. Ambulatory surgical centers will start to enroll within the next year. Currently, community outpatient imaging centers that are not affiliated with an acute-care hospital are unable to participate in the program. To participate, one

Table 2
Six domains for OIE measure categorization

Domain	Description
Duplication	Studies that are duplicated within a short time of each other without any identified clinical indication
Overlap	Different imaging modalities for the same area of the body within a short time of each other that serve the same clinical purpose
Screening	Imaging studies without identified clinical indications based on symptoms or existing diagnoses
Negative studies	Clinically noncontributory studies
With and without contrast	Imaging studies repeated in a short timeframe on same body area differing only in whether contrast is used
Adjacent body areas	Imaging studies repeated in a short timeframe on adjacent body areas

Data from Centers for Medicare and Medicare Services. Outpatient imaging efficiency measures. Available at: http:// hospitaloqr.com/media/HandoutsImagingMeasuresNotePages.pdf.

Table 3
Selection criteria for OIE measures

Criterion	Description
Importance and relevance	In respect to prevalence, cost burden, and vulnerable populations
Scientific soundness	Consistent with evidence-based clinical guidelines
Usability	Clear guidelines that highlight room for improvement
Feasibility	Minimal data collection requirements

Data from QualityNet. Imaging efficiency measures. Available at: http://www.qualitynet.org.

must complete the registration process for outpatient hospitals at http://www.qualitynet.org.[14] In 2010, there were 3394 total HOP QDRP eligible hospitals.[15] Of these, 3288 met the requirements to receive the full APU under HOPPS. Eleven hospitals failed to meet the requirements, and 95 chose not to participate.

Resources

More information about HOP QDRP, its payment plan, and OIE measures can be found at the CMS Web site: https://www.cms.gov/HospitalQuality Inits/10_HospitalOutpatientQualityReportingProgram. asp.[16] A brief synopsis of HOP QDRP is in press in the *American Journal of Neuroradiology*.[17] Publications by the Institute of Medicine[18] and Bentley and coworkers[19] provide additional resources for defining waste in health care.

HOSPITAL OUTPATIENT PROSPECTIVE PAYMENT SYSTEM
Overview

A brief review of HOPPS is provided highlighting the program's legislative history, outpatient service classifications, and payment plan. Specifically, how HOPPS is relevant for the practicing radiologist is discussed. Resources are also provided for further information on the program details and the ambulatory payment classifications (APC) system.

History and Background

HOPPS is a payment system, established in August 2000 by government legislation,[20] replacing the existing fee-for-service system and is currently used by CMS to reimburse for hospital outpatient services. Hospitals receive a 2% reduction in their APU under the HOPPS program for not successfully meeting the requirements of HOP QDRP, a financial incentive program for hospitals

to meet certain quality control criteria in the outpatient setting. Please refer to the previous section for further information on HOP QDRP.

The HOPPS program was developed in response to the growing need for a prospective payment system. In 1965, the Medicare program retrospectively reimbursed medical services on the basis of hospital-specific reasonable costs.[21] As a result of this system and a Medicare-driven increase in demand for medical services, healthcare costs increased markedly. The federal government responded in 1983 by creating a hospital inpatient prospective payment system, better known as the diagnosis-related grouping (DRG) system. The DRG system established a fixed prospectively determined payment structure based on patient diagnosis that reimbursed all products and services used to treat a given diagnosis with a single payment. The DRG system also shifted inpatient costs in excess of the fixed payment to the hospital itself rather than to Medicare. This placed the financial risk associated with extended patient stays on hospitals as an incentive to promote efficient use of healthcare resources and provide less costly care. Outpatient services, which were not part of the DRG system, continued to be reimbursed with cost taken into account. This led to higher billing charges and led to the establishment of the current HOPPS. Thus, similar to the DRG system for inpatient usage, HOPPS is intended to control healthcare costs through a prospective bundled payment system. This program is complex, and represents a challenge for the radiology community to understand and use the new system.

Ambulatory Payment Classifications

APC is the grouping system developed for reimbursing the provision of hospital outpatient services, including outpatient imaging. All covered outpatient services are assigned to an APC group. Each group of procedure codes within an APC is clinically similar with regards to resource consumption. There are five composite APCs for imaging services: (1) ultrasound, (2) CT and CT angiography without contrast, (3) CT and CT angiography with contrast, (4) MR imaging and MR angiography without contrast, and (5) MR imaging and MR angiography with contrast.[22] For example, in the APC 8007 group (MR imaging and MR angiography without contrast) there are 26 coded procedures including MR imaging and MR angiography without contrast of all body parts, such as brain, chest, and extremities. The payment rate and copayment calculated for an APC apply to each service within the APC as shown in **Table 5**.

Table 4
HOP QDRP measures applicable to radiology

Number	Name	Description
OP-8	MR imaging lumbar spine for low back pain	The percentage of patients who had MR imaging of the lumbar spine with a diagnosis of low back pain without Medicare claims-based evidence of antecedent conservative therapy.
OP-9	Mammography follow-up rates	The percentage of patients with mammography screening studies done in the outpatient hospital setting that are followed within 45 days by diagnostic mammography or ultrasound of the breast in an outpatient or office setting.
OP-10	Abdomen CT: use of contrast material	The ratio of CT abdomen studies that are performed with and without contrast out of all CT abdomen studies performed (those with contrast, those without contrast, and those with both).
OP-11	Thorax CT: use of contrast material	The ratio of CT thorax studies that are performed with and without contrast out of all CT thorax studies performed (those with contrast, those without contrast, and those with both).
OP-13	Cardiac imaging for preoperative risk assessment for noncardiac, low-risk surgery	The ratio of stress echocardiography, single-photon emission CT myocardial perfusion imaging, and stress MR imaging studies performed within 30 days of ambulatory, low-risk, noncardiac surgery out of the total number of outpatient studies performed. High values may indicate high use of stress tests before low-risk, noncardiac procedures and raise the question of inefficient examination protocols.
OP-14	Simultaneous use of brain CT and sinus CT	The percentage of brain CT studies that are simultaneously accompanied by a sinus CT study. High values may indicate high use of simultaneous brain and sinus CT examinations and raise the question of inefficient examination protocols and exposure to additional unnecessary radiation.
OP-15	Use of brain CT in the emergency department for atraumatic headache	This measure calculates the percentage of emergency department visits with a coincident brain CT study out of all emergency department visits with a primary diagnosis of headache. High values may indicate high use of brain CT in the emergency department for atraumatic headache and raise the question of inefficient clinical examination protocols.

Data from Centers for Medicare and Medicare Services. Outpatient imaging efficiency measures. Available at: http://hospitaloqr.com/media/HandoutsImagingMeasuresNotePages.pdf.

Although each outpatient procedure group has a single APC rate, this does not translate to equal reimbursement for identical services. Surgical rates are subject to discounting when multiple procedures are performed contemporaneously, with the most expensive APC group paid in full and all other groups paid at half of their APC rate. However, at this time radiology procedures are not yet subject to this provision.

Payment System

The payment rate for most medical and surgical services is calculated by multiplying the

Table 5
Example of the HOPPS list of APCs with SI, relative weights, and copayment amounts in 2007

APC Group	Group Title	SI	Relative Weight	Payment Rate	National Unadjusted Copayment	Minimum Unadjusted Copayment
0272	Fluoroscopy	X	1.2908	79.34	31.64	15.87
0274	Myelography	S	2.5544	157.01	62.80	31.40
0279	Level II angiography and venography	S	9.5061	584.32	150.03	116.86
0280	Level III angiography and venography	S	20.8225	1279.92	353.85	255.98
0282	Miscellaneous computerized axial tomography	S	1.5379	94.53	37.81	18.91
0283	CT with contrast	S	4.0825	250.94	100.37	50.19
0284	MR imaging and MR angiography with contrast	S	6.1231	376.37	148.40	75.27
0296	Level II therapeutic radiologic procedures	S	2.6802	164.75	53.99	32.95
0297	Level III therapeutic radiologic procedures	S	3.6392	223.69	89.47	44.74
0298	Level IV therapeutic radiologic procedures	S	8.3906	515.75	206.30	103.15
0332	CT without contrast	S	3.0908	189.99	75.24	38.00
0333	CT without contrast followed by contrast	S	4.8405	297.54	119.01	59.51
0335	MR imaging, miscellaneous	S	4.5523	279.82	111.92	55.96
0336	MR imaging and MR angiography without contrast	S	5.6745	348.80	139.51	69.76
0337	MR imaging and MR angiography without contrast followed by contrast	S	8.1155	498.84	199.53	99.77

Abbreviations: APC, ambulatory payment classifications; S, significant procedure, not discounted when multiple; SI, status indicator; X, ancillary services.
Data from Centers for Medicare and Medicare Services. Available at: http://www.cms.gov/Medicare/Medicare-Fee-for-Service-Payment/HospitalOutpatientPPS/downloads//CMS1506FC.pdf.

prospectively established scaled relative weight for the service's clinical APC by a conversion factor to determine the national unadjusted payment rate for the APC. The scaled relative weight for an APC measures the resource requirements of the service and is based on the median cost of services in that APC group. The conversion factor translates the scaled relative weights into dollar payment rates.[23] To account for geographic differences in input prices, the labor portion of the national unadjusted payment rate (60%) is further adjusted by multiplying by the hospital wage index for the area in which the hospital is located. The remaining 40% is not adjusted.[23] For example, the national unadjusted payment rate for APC code 0336, MR imaging and MR angiography without contrast, is 139.45. The labor portion of this is 139.51 * 0.6 = 83.76 and the nonlabor portion is 139.51 * 0.4 = 55.80. In Lawton, Oklahoma, which has the lowest geographic wage index of 0.7666, the adjusted labor portion is 83.76 * 0.7666 = 64.21. When added to the nonlabor portion, the national adjusted payment is 64.21 + 55.80 = 120.014. However, the highest geographic wage index is in Oakland-Fremont-Hayward, California, with a wage index of 1.5436. Doing a similar calculation, the national adjusted payment becomes 83.76 * 1.5436 + 55.80 = 185.09. Therefore, the national adjusted payment for MR imaging and MR angiography without contrast examinations varies from 120.01 to 185.09 according to geographic areas in the United States.

Several factors were considered in the establishment of APC reimbursement rates. Initially, CMS used fiscal-year 1996 outpatient claims cost data for specific procedures as a basis for reimbursement, with data to be updated annually. Additional considerations in the reimbursement are other expenses incurred in the furnishing of services, such as anesthesia and anesthesia recovery costs, supplies, capital expenses, and costs to procure donor tissue. The cost of drugs and biologics are incorporated into the APC system, although some new drugs may be eligible for special transitional pass-through payments. There are also specific exceptions for certain items, such as corneal tissue acquisition, blood and blood products, casting and splints, immunosuppressive drugs for organ transplantation, and other similarly and infrequently used drugs.[24]

Congress has allowed some additional sources of reimbursement through the Balanced Budget Refinement Act.[25] Initially, the act provides pass-through payments for new drugs, devices, and biologics during the first 2 to 3 years that the product is on the market. In addition, transitional-corridor payments were added to compensate for patients with unusual expenses or for hospital costs that exceeded the APC rate. Finally, CMS created a special group of new-technology APCs for new services or procedures. As a result of these additional provisions, HOPPS has become an extensive, complex mechanism for hospital and physician reimbursement, and will likely continue to undergo change to meet future challenges of the healthcare system.

Resources

More information about the HOPPS program, APCs, and payment system can be found at the CMS Web site: https://www.cms.gov/Hospital OutpatientPPS/. A brief synopsis of the HOPPS program is in press in the *American Journal of Neuroradiology*.[26,27]

REFERENCES

1. Tax Relief and Health Care Act of 2006, Bill No. H.R. 61111, Public Law No. 109–432, Title I, §101.
2. Medicare, Medicaid, and State Children's Health Insurance Program Extension Act of 2007, Bill No. S.2499, Public Law No. 110–173, Title I, §131.
3. Medicare Improvements for Patients and Providers Act of 2003, Bill No. H.R. 6331, Public Law No. 110–275, Title I, §131.
4. Affordable Care Act of 2010, Bill No. H.R. 3590, Public Law No. 111–148, Title III, §3002.
5. Available at: http://www.acr.org/SecondaryMainMenu Categories/quality_safety/p4p/FeaturedCategories/P4P Initiatives/pqri/FeaturedCategories/resources/PQRS-2012-Update-Final.aspx. Accessed January 5, 2012.
6. Available at: http://www.acr.org/SecondaryMainMenu Categories/quality_safety/p4p/FeaturedCategories/P4P Initiatives/pqri/FeaturedCategories/resources/Validation ofSuccessfulReporting/MAVFlowchart.aspx. Accessed January 5, 2012.
7. Available at: http://www.cms.gov/Medicare/Quality-Initiatives-Patient-Assessment-Instruments/PQRS/down loads//2011_PhysQualRptg_MeasureSpecifications Manual_033111.pdf. Accessed January 5, 2012.
8. Available at: https://www.cms.gov/Medicare/Quality-Initiatives-Patient-Assessment-Instruments/PQRS/How_ To_Get_Started.html. Accessed January 5, 2012.
9. Services (CMS) website. Available at: www.cms.hhs. gov/PQRS. Includes information on eligibility criteria, reporting measures, and reporting statistics by year and specialty. Accessed January 5, 2012.
10. Anumula N, Sanelli PC. Physician Quality Reporting System. AJNR Am J Neuroradiol 2011;32(11):2000–1.
11. Hospital Compare website. Available at: www.hospi talcompare.hhs.gov. Accessed January 5, 2012.

12. Available at: https://www.cms.gov/Medicare/Quality-Initiatives-Patient-Assessment-Instruments/Hospital QualityInits/HospitalOutpatientQualityReportingProgram.html. Accessed January 5, 2012.

13. Available at: https://www.cms.gov/HospitalQuality Inits/Downloads/HospitalOutpatientImagingEfficiency MinimumCaseCounts.pdf. Accessed January 5, 2012.

14. Available at: http://www.qualitynet.org. Accessed January 5, 2012.

15. Available at: https://www.cms.gov/Medicare/Quality-Initiatives-Patient-Assessment-Instruments/Hospital QualityInits/Downloads/Archived-data-from-January-1-2010-to-Dec-31-2010.zip. Accessed January 5, 2012.

16. Available at: https://www.cms.gov/HospitalQuality Inits/10_HospitalOutpatientQualityReportingProgram.asp. Accessed January 5, 2012.

17. Anumula N, Sanelli PC. Hospital outpatient quality data reporting program. AJNR Am J Neuroradiol 2012;33(2):225–6.

18. Institute of Medicine. Committee on Quality of Health Care in America. Crossing the Quality Chasm: a new health system for the 21st century. Washington, DC: National Academies Press; 2001.

19. Bentley TG, Effros RM, Palar K, et al. Waste in the U.S. health care system: a conceptual framework. Milbank Q 2008;86:629–59.

20. Social Security Act, P. L. 74-271 Title 18 §1833; Balanced Budget Act, P.L. 74-271, H.R. 2015, Title IV.

21. Health Insurance for the Aged of 1965, Pub L No. 89-97; 79 Stat 291; 42 USC §102.

22. Available at: http://www.cms.gov/Regulations-and-Guidance/Guidance/Transmittals/downloads//R2141CP.pdf. Accessed January 5, 2012.

23. Available at: https://www.cms.gov/Outreach-and-Education/Medicare-Learning-Network-MLN/MLN Products/downloads//HospitalOutpaysysfctsht.pdf. Accessed January 5, 2012.

24. Smith JJ, Maida A, Henderson JA, et al. Hospital outpatient prospective payment under Medicare: understanding the system and its implications. Radiology 2002;225:13–9.

25. Balanced Budget Refinement Act, Bill No. H.R. 3426, Public Law No. 106–113, Title II, §1.

26. Available at: https://www.cms.gov/HospitalOutpatient PPS/. Accessed January 5, 2012.

27. Anumula N, Sanelli PC. Hospital outpatient prospective payment system. AJNR Am J Neuroradiol 2012;33(4):616.

Evidence-Based Imaging and Effective Utilization
Lessons in Neuroradiology

Francisco A. Perez, MD, PhD[a],
Jeffrey G. Jarvik, MD, MPH[b,c,d,e,f],*

KEYWORDS

• Neuroradiology • Evidence-based imaging • Comparative effectiveness • Utilization

KEY POINTS

- Overutilization of imaging contributes to increasing health care costs.
- Evidence-based imaging decreases costs and improves outcomes by guiding appropriate utilization of imaging.
- Although evidence-based imaging guidelines recommend against the use of early magnetic resonance (MR) imaging for uncomplicated low back pain, spine MR imaging utilization has increased, often inappropriately.
- Barriers to practicing evidence-based imaging, such as in low back pain, include patient- and physician-related factors.
- Overcoming barriers to practicing evidence-based imaging requires leadership by radiologists.

GROWTH OF MEDICAL IMAGING

Medical costs in the United States continue to exceed 17% of the Gross Domestic Product each year or more than $2 trillion, greater than any other country.[1] Although computed tomography (CT) and magnetic resonance (MR) imaging are ranked by physicians as the most important innovation to affect their patients,[2] have been recognized through Nobel prizes, and are often celebrated when new units are opened in a community,[3] the proliferation of advanced imaging, more than double the number of units from 2000 to 2008,[1] comes at a high cost. Imaging is one the largest drivers of increasing medical costs. From 1998 to 2005, among Medicare patients the compound annual growth rate for diagnostic imaging was 4.1%.[4] From 2000 to 2009, volume growth of imaging for Medicare patients grew 85%, nearly double the rate for all physician services.[5] For example, in neuroimaging, the volume of spine MR imaging performed for Medicare patients in the private office setting tripled from 1998 to 2008, greater than that for head MR imaging (Fig. 1).[6]

Disclosures: Jeffrey G. Jarvik is a Member of Comparative Effectiveness Research Advisory Board of GE Healthcare, Stockholder and Co-founder of PhysioSonics and Consultant to HealthHelp.
[a] Department of Radiology, School of Medicine, University of Washington, Box 357115, 1959 Northeast Pacific Street, Room RR215, Seattle, WA 98195-7115, USA; [b] Department of Radiology, Harborview Medical Center, School of Medicine, University of Washington, Box 359728, 325 Ninth Avenue, Seattle, WA 98104-2499, USA; [c] Comparative Effectiveness, Cost and Outcomes Research Center, University of Washington, Box 359728, 325 Ninth Ave, Seattle, WA 98104, USA; [d] Department of Neurological Surgery, School of Medicine, University of Washington, 325 Ninth Ave, Seattle, WA 98104, USA; [e] Department of Health Services, School of Public Health, University of Washington, 1959 NE Pacific St, Seattle, WA 98195, USA; [f] School of Pharmacy, Box 357631, 1959 NE Pacific St, Seattle, WA 98195, USA
* Corresponding author. Department of Radiology, School of Medicine, Harborview Medical Center, University of Washington, Box 359728, 325 Ninth Avenue, Seattle, WA 98104-2499.
E-mail address: jarvikj@uw.edu

Neuroimag Clin N Am 22 (2012) 467–476
doi:10.1016/j.nic.2012.05.002

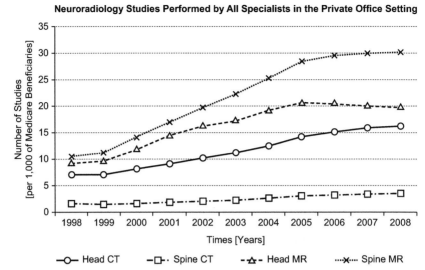

Fig. 1. Growth of neuroimaging for outpatient Medicare patients. (*Reproduced from* Babiarz LS, Yousem DM, Parker L, et al. Utilization rates of neuroradiology across neuroscience specialties in the private office setting: who owns or leases the scanners on which studies are performed? AJNR Am J Neuroradiol 2012;33(1):43–8; © American Society of Neuroradiology; with permission.)

This increased utilization and growth of medical imaging is financially unsustainable. Most importantly, approximately 30% of advanced imaging is likely inappropriate[7,8] and could account for $40 billion of the $480 billion in excess health care expenditures in the United States compared with other countries.[9]

In addition to financial costs of unnecessary imaging, there are health costs including radiation exposure in the case of CT scanning and radiography, associated increased cancer risk,[10] and the consequences of incidental findings. Inappropriate imaging often results in undesirable additional testing and invasive procedures, resulting not only in increased costs but also worse outcomes. Practicing evidence-based imaging can guide appropriate use of imaging, decrease unnecessary imaging-related health care costs, and reduce unnecessary risks to patients.

LOW BACK PAIN: AN OPPORTUNITY FOR EFFECTIVE IMAGING UTILIZATION

Low back pain is one of the most common reasons for visits to primary care physicians, with estimated direct medical costs of over $80 billion in 2005.[11] Moreover, the costs of health care related to back pain continue to increase without evidence of a corresponding improvement in self-assessed health status.[11] Part of these escalating costs are due to frequent imaging of patients with back pain, including expensive lumbar spine MR imaging. Given overall increasing health care expenditures, low back pain has been an

appropriate target for effectiveness research over the past 2 decades. Appropriate utilization of imaging for low back pain can be optimized by applying evidence-based imaging methods, particularly in the context of comparative-effectiveness research studies, to a technology assessment framework.

Evidence-Based Imaging for Low Back Pain

Evidence-based imaging involves formulating a clinical question, identifying the relevant medical literature, assessing the literature, summarizing the data, and then applying the evidence to make an appropriate clinical decision. Evidence from the most reliable research can be integrated with a physician's expertise and the patient's expectations to guide medical decision making regarding which, if any, imaging study is appropriate for a given clinical question.[12] In the context of low back pain, a specific evidence-based clinical question relevant to appropriate utilization would be: in a patient with acute low back pain without evidence of cauda equina syndrome or concern for systemic disease, is early (within 4–6 weeks of symptom onset) lumbar spine MR imaging an effective and appropriate strategy? When evaluating this question, one should use the highest-quality research available, such as prospective, randomized controlled trials, to reduce the potential for bias. Fortunately, there is a reasonable amount of high-quality research focused on low back pain.

Comparative-effectiveness research studies are particularly useful in evaluating appropriate utilization of imaging because they compare the effectiveness, benefits, and harms of existing diagnostic imaging tests. Moreover, differences in the costs of care between the imaging technologies compared are often simultaneously addressed as part of a cost-outcomes study. For example, Jarvik and colleagues[13] conducted a randomized, prospective study in patients with uncomplicated low back pain in a primary care setting by comparing the impact of early lumbar spine MR imaging versus radiographs on disability, pain, preference scores, satisfaction, and costs. Both groups demonstrated improvements in several measures of low back pain disability and pain over time consistent with the natural history of uncomplicated low back pain. Although patients and physicians preferred rapid MR imaging over radiographs, there was no long-term difference in disability, pain, or general health. On the other hand, there was a nonsignificant trend toward increased spine surgery in patients undergoing early MR imaging as well as associated increased costs.

In another randomized, prospective study evaluating outcomes and cost-effectiveness of imaging for low back pain in the primary care setting, Gilbert and colleagues[14] compared the use of early, nonselective MR imaging or CT imaging versus delayed MR imaging or CT in select patients who developed a clear clinical need for imaging. Clinical treatments were similar in both groups, with improvements in back pain; however, there were slightly greater improvements in low back pain and quality-adjusted life year

(QALY) estimates with early imaging, which was of questionable clinical significance. Measuring QALY, an indicator of disease burden including both quantity and quality of life, in combination with cost data allows for evaluation of the cost-effectiveness of the 2 imaging strategies. With this information, one can determine whether the additional costs justify the potential small benefit.

Comprehensive Technology Assessment of MR Imaging for Low Back Pain

Whereas evidence-based medicine provides the tools for evaluating evidence related to effective utilization of imaging, technology assessment provides a framework to critically evaluate the comprehensive performance of imaging technologies by addressing a hierarchy of specific questions for a given patient population (for a detailed review see Hollingworth and Jarvik[15]). For a given technology, such as MR imaging for evaluation of low back pain, the hierarchy of technology-assessment questions that can be addressed using the evidence-based medicine process are outlined in **Table 1**.[16]

In the context of uncomplicated acute low back pain, there have been many studies that have evaluated these questions for lumbar spine MR imaging. For example, with regard to diagnostic performance and impact, many MR imaging findings, including loss of disc height, disc protrusions, and annular fissures, are so common in patients without back pain that they are nonspecific. Disc extrusions, on the other hand, are uncommon in an asymptomatic population and could be more likely to account for low back

Table 1
Comprehensive technology assessment of MR imaging for low back pain

Factor	Questions
Technical performance	Are the images from a lumbar spine MR imaging technically adequate to reliably evaluate anatomy?
Diagnostic performance	Can an accurate diagnosis be made from the MR imaging images? What are the interobserver and intraobserver reliability? What imaging findings on lumbar spine MR imaging could account for causes of low back pain?
Diagnostic impact	Does the use of lumbar spine MR imaging change the diagnostic confidence or the use of other testing when evaluating the cause of low back pain?
Therapeutic impact	Does lumbar spine MR imaging change clinical management in a patient with low back pain?
Health impact	Does the use of lumbar spine MR imaging affect the outcomes of a patient with low back pain?
Societal impact	Is the use of lumbar spine MR imaging cost-effective?

pain.[17] The evaluation of therapeutic impact of lumbar spine MR imaging for uncomplicated low back pain, as defined in Table 1, is often negative because it can lead to unnecessary surgery,[13,18] as most patients will improve without intervention and regardless of whether they receive advanced imaging.[19] With regard to the health-impact assessment of lumbar spine MR imaging, a patient's knowledge of nonspecific imaging findings on lumbar spine MR imaging, such as disc protrusions, could negatively affect a patient's overall sense of well-being.[20] On the other hand, early lumbar spine MR imaging may lead to a slightly greater improvement in pain in comparison with no or late imaging.[14] At a societal level, early lumbar spine MR imaging in the absence of "red flags" for serious conditions is unlikely to be cost-effective.[14]

By applying evidence-based imaging methods to a series of hierarchical questions in this abbreviated example of technology assessment, early MR imaging in uncomplicated back pain does not improve outcomes, leads to increased costs, and can cause negative outcomes such as radiation exposure, for example from additional testing with CT or radiographs, and unnecessary procedures.

SUMMARY EVIDENCE-BASED RESOURCES

Finding and evaluating evidence-based medicine methods can be time consuming, particularly when there is an extensive body of primary research literature such as for imaging in low back pain. Summary evidence-based resources, such as systematic reviews, appropriateness criteria, and clinical guidelines, are tools that summarize and evaluate the supporting evidence to facilitate the practice of evidence-based imaging and effective utilization.

Systematic Reviews and Meta-Analysis

Systematic reviews aim to reduce bias when evaluating a specific topic by using the evidence-based medicine process to exhaustively identify, assess, summarize, and synthesize findings from all relevant studies. Using specialized statistical methods, primary data from selected studies can be synthesized quantitatively as part of a meta-analysis to evaluate potential bias and increase statistical power. For example, Chou and colleagues[21] conducted a systematic review and meta-analysis to evaluate the use of early imaging for low back pain in patients without indication of serious underlying conditions versus usual clinical care without early imaging. Their literature searches identified more than 450 potentially

relevant articles; on further assessment of these articles, 6 randomized trials of sufficient quality were identified comparing early imaging using radiographs, CT, and/or MR imaging versus no early imaging in the evaluation of low back pain. A meta-analysis was then performed by combining the primary data from several of these 6 studies. The investigators found that early imaging does not improve short-term or long-term outcomes for pain, function, quality of life, mental health, or a measure of overall improvement in the health of patients with uncomplicated low back pain.

Appropriateness Criteria

Whereas systematic reviews and meta-analysis help to facilitate the process for evaluating effective use of imaging by synthesizing a large body of evidence, appropriateness criteria and clinical guidelines provide more practical recommendations regarding effective use of imaging.

The American College of Radiology (ACR) Appropriateness Criteria were first developed in the early 1990s to help guide the appropriate use of imaging. There are currently 17 major neuroradiologic imaging topics (Box 1) that are addressed

---

Box 1
Available ACR neuroradiology appropriateness criteria

- Ataxia
- Cerebrovascular disease
- Cranial neuropathy
- Dementia and movement disorders
- Focal neurologic deficit
- Head trauma
- Headache
- Low back pain
- Myelopathy
- Neck mass/adenopathy
- Neuroendocrine imaging
- Orbits, vision, and visual loss
- Plexopathy
- Seizures and epilepsy
- Sinonasal disease
- Suspected spine trauma
- Vertigo and hearing loss

Data from ACR. ACR Appropriateness Criteria. Available at: http://www.acr.org/ac. Accessed January 7, 2012.

including low back pain, headache, and head trauma. For each of these larger topics, the guidelines are further subdivided into various clinical scenarios. For example, in low back pain 6 clinical variants are addressed, as outlined in **Box 2**. For each of these clinical scenarios different radiological procedures, such as MR imaging, CT, myelography, radiography, and bone scans, are rated on a scale of 1 to 9 based on their determined appropriateness, with 9 being "usually appropriate."[22] A committee of experts assigns appropriateness ratings based on individual interpretations of the relevant literature until consensus is reached using a modified Delphi technique.[23] In the case of uncomplicated, acute low back pain, without red flags to suggest more serious causes of low back pain, as defined in **Box 3**, all reviewed imaging modalities, including lumbar spine MR imaging, were rated a 2 and considered "usually not appropriate." On the other hand, when systemic disease such as infection or cancer is suspected, lumbar spine MR imaging is rated an 8 and considered "usually appropriate"[22]; the appropriateness ratings for other imaging tests in this clinical scenario are summarized in **Fig. 2**.

Clinical Guidelines

Clinical guidelines gather, critically appraise, and synthesize the evidence, and make actionable recommendations relevant to a clinical question. Whereas ACR Appropriateness Criteria assist in determining which imaging study is most appropriate in a specific clinical scenario, clinical guidelines are more encompassing and help determine which patients should undergo imaging as well as initial management. As with appropriateness criteria, clinical guidelines are often developed using a committee approach relying on

---

> **Box 2**
> **ACR Appropriateness Criteria clinical variants for low back pain**
>
> - Uncomplicated, acute low back pain
> - Low-velocity trauma, osteoporosis, or age greater than 70 years
> - Suspicion of cancer, infection, or immunosuppression
> - Low back pain and/or radiculopathy in surgical or interventional candidate
> - Prior lumbar surgery
> - Cauda equina syndrome
>
> *Data from* Davis PC, Wippold FJ 2nd, Brunberg JA, et al. ACR Appropriateness Criteria on low back pain. J Am Coll Radiol 2009;6(6):401–7.

> **Box 3**
> **ACR Appropriateness Criteria red flags indicating complicated low back pain**
>
> - Recent significant trauma, or milder trauma, age greater than 50 years
> - Unexplained weight loss
> - Unexplained fever
> - Immunosuppression
> - History of cancer
> - Intravenous drug use
> - Prolonged use of corticosteroids, osteoporosis
> - Age greater than 70 years
> - Focal neurologic deficit with progressive or disabling symptoms
> - Duration longer than 6 weeks
>
> *Data from* Davis PC, Wippold FJ 2nd, Brunberg JA, et al. ACR Appropriateness Criteria on low back pain. J Am Coll Radiol 2009;6(6):401–7.

---

a combination of systematic reviews, when available, as well as expert opinion. For example, the American College of Physicians and American Pain Society[24] have developed clinical guidelines for the diagnosis and treatment of low back pain. Using a technology-assessment paradigm and relying on systematic reviews and meta-analyses, such as the one described by Chou and colleagues,[21] the guidelines provide evidence-based recommendations as to which patients with low back pain should be imaged, with which modality, and when they should be imaged (see **Box 4** for a summary of recommendations related to lumbar spine MR imaging). One of their recommendations is that "Clinicians should not routinely obtain imaging or other diagnostic tests in patients with nonspecific low back pain (strong recommendation, moderate-quality evidence)." As with many clinical guidelines, the strength of a recommendation as well as the quality of the evidence underlying the recommendation are graded.

EVIDENCE IS NOT SUFFICIENT: BARRIERS TO PRACTICING EVIDENCE-BASED IMAGING

Uncomplicated acute low back pain is a unique example for which there is adequate literature, including randomized controlled trials and meta-analysis, evaluating the clinical and cost-effectiveness of various imaging strategies. Despite the overwhelming evidence and clinical guidelines demonstrating that early imaging with MR for uncomplicated low back pain leads to

Clinical Condition: Low Back Pain

Variant 3:   Patient with one or more of the following: suspicion of cancer, infection, and/or immunosuppression.

Radiologic Procedure	Rating	Comments	RRL*
MRI lumbar spine without and with contrast	8	Contrast useful for neoplasia subjects suspected of epidural or intraspinal disease. See statement regarding contrast in text under "Anticipated Exceptions."	O
MRI lumbar spine without contrast	7	Noncontrast MRI may be sufficient if there is low risk of epidural and/or intraspinal disease.	O
CT lumbar spine with contrast	6	MRI preferred. CT useful if MRI is contraindicated or unavailable, and/or for problem solving.	☢☢☢
CT lumbar spine without contrast	6	MRI preferred. CT useful if MRI is contraindicated or unavailable, and/or for problem solving.	☢☢☢
X-ray lumbar spine	5		☢☢☢
Tc-99m bone scan whole body with SPECT spine	5	SPECT/CT may be useful for anatomic localization and problem solving.	☢☢☢
X-ray myelography lumbar spine	2		☢☢☢
Myelography and postmyelography CT lumbar spine	2	In some cases postinjection CT imaging may be done without plain-film myelography.	☢☢☢☢

Rating Scale: 1,2,3 Usually not appropriate; 4,5,6 May be appropriate; 7,8,9 Usually appropriate   *Relative Radiation Level

Fig. 2. ACR Appropriateness Criteria for low back pain with suspicion of cancer, infection, or immunosuppression. (*Reprinted from* American College of Radiology. No other representation of this material is authorized without expressed, written permission from the American College of Radiology. Refer to the ACR Web site at www.acr.org/ac for the most current and complete version of the ACR Appropriateness Criteria®[23]; with permission.)

increased costs without significant clinical benefit, the use of MR imaging for low back pain continues to increase. For example, although clinical guidelines from as early as 1994 recommended against routine use of imaging in evaluation of uncomplicated low back pain,[25] spine MR imaging utilization has increased at a compound annual growth rate of approximately 11% from 1998 to 2008,

---

Box 4
Summary of American College of Physicians clinical guidelines for MR imaging in low back pain

- Immediate MR imaging of lumbar spine if risk factors for or signs of spinal infection, cauda equina syndrome, or severe neurologic deficits

- MR imaging of lumbar spine after a trial of therapy if signs or symptoms of radiculopathy or spinal stenosis in patients who are candidates for surgical intervention

Data from Chou R, Qaseem A, Owens DK, et al. Diagnostic imaging for low back pain: advice for high-value health care from the American College of Physicians. Ann Intern Med 2011;154(3):181–9.

---

which is greater than that for other neuroradiology procedures including head CT or head MR imaging.[6] At the authors' academic center, 35% of outpatient spine MR imaging studies ordered by primary care physicians were considered inappropriate.[7] Even after introduction of clinical guidelines at another institution, Williams and colleagues[26] found no change in the management of patients and specifically no difference in the utilization of imaging for evaluation of new episodes of low back pain among general practitioners in a primary care setting. In other words, inappropriate utilization of advanced imaging for low back pain continues because evidence-based imaging and clinical guidelines, even when they are well worked out, are not being practiced.

Understanding the barriers to adopting and adhering to the practice of evidence-based imaging is critical for realizing the potential benefits of comparative-effectiveness research. Many of the barriers are listed in Table 2, and some of these barriers are addressed in detail by other articles in this issue. To effect change in imaging utilization, ultimately patients and physicians must recognize and overcome their barriers to adopting evidenced-based imaging.

Table 2
Barriers to practicing evidence-based imaging and potential solutions

Barrier	Solutions
Lack of awareness of clinical guidelines and appropriateness criteria	Clinician education including by radiologists
Numerous, constantly updating clinical guidelines	Systematic reviews of guidelines Coordination and consolidation of clinical guideline creation Decision support tools Radiology benefits management Clinician education including by radiologists
Lack of evidence	Funding for comparative-effectiveness research Comparative-effectiveness research by radiologists
Self-referral financial incentives	Health care reform Legislation to prohibit self-referral Radiology benefits management Decision support tools
Fee-for-service financial incentives	Health care reform Managed care Accountable care organizations Value-based reimbursements Bundled payments Radiology benefits management Decision support Radiologist consultations
Patient expectations for imaging studies to be performed	Patient education by clinicians and radiologists Increased patient cost sharing
Fear of potential litigation	Tort reform

Patient Barriers to Practicing Evidence-Based Imaging

Patients are skeptical of evidence-based medicine and imaging. There is a public perception that care relying on costly, newer technologies is of superior quality whereas less expensive care is lower quality.[27] In addition, physician practice, including ineffective use of imaging, can be influenced by patients' requests.[28] Patients expect imaging as part of their evaluation to identify a cause for their back pain.[29,30] Moreover, when more expensive imaging such as MR imaging rather than radiography is used, patients with low back pain are more satisfied.[13] The overuse of imaging in low back pain and other conditions could be driven by a need-to-know mentality.[31] For example, some physicians knowingly obtain "inappropriate" imaging to reassure patients, particularly when patients request imaging studies.[32]

Physician Barriers to Practicing Evidence-Based Imaging

At a basic level, many physicians do not practice evidence-based imaging because they are unaware of clinical guidelines and appropriateness criteria. For example, Bautista and colleagues[33] found in a survey that almost no referring physicians used the ACR Appropriateness Criteria as one of their top 3 resources when determining the most appropriate imaging study for a patient; they preferred radiologist consultation, specialty journals, and UpToDate. On the other hand, physicians who are aware of clinical guidelines may be overwhelmed by the sheer number of different clinical guidelines and the frequency with which they are updated. For example, a systematic review of clinical guidelines for the management of low back pain identified nearly 100 relevant clinical guidelines since 2000.[34]

Physicians are financially rewarded for not practicing evidence-based imaging, particularly when they own the imaging equipment. In the current United States fee-for-service health care payment system they are compensated for performing imaging studies, regardless of their appropriateness. In 2001, self-referral was estimated to account for $16 billion of inappropriate imaging.[35] Babiarz and colleagues[6] recently demonstrated that the growth of utilization rates for advanced neuroimaging in the private office setting was highest among nonradiologist groups, such as neurosurgeons and other specialty groups, who owned or leased their own equipment. Specifically for low back pain, self-referring physicians use imaging at a rate 5 times higher than do radiologist-referring physicians.[36]

Fear of litigation and the practice of defensive medicine are additional reasons why physicians may not practice evidence-based imaging. In the United States the medical liability system, including costs related to defensive medicine, have been estimated to account for at least $56 billion or 2.4% of total health care spending in 2008.[37] Surveys of malpractice litigation identify an increasing number of cases whereby there was a failure to order an imaging study.[38] Because clinical guidelines cannot be 100% sensitive, there will be cases whereby an imaging study is not performed based on evidence-based criteria but a critical diagnosis is missed or delayed, resulting in patient harm. Punishing the physician who practiced evidence-based imaging in such cases will motivate physicians to practice defensive medicine in favor of effective utilization.

SOLUTIONS FOR IMPROVING THE PRACTICE OF EVIDENCE-BASED IMAGING

To achieve effective utilization of imaging, the barriers to the practice of evidence-based imaging need to be addressed. This action requires a multifactorial approach including modification of financial incentives, physician behavior, and patient expectations. This approach is summarized in **Table 2** and is covered in more detail in other articles in this issue.

One strategy to overcome the barriers of practicing evidence-based imaging is to use systems, rather than relying on individual ordering physicians, to determine the appropriateness of an imaging study. For example, radiology benefits management programs and decision support systems aim to influence patient imaging requests on a case-by-case assessment of appropriateness before approval (see the article by Yousem elsewhere in this issue). For management of radiology utilization, a referring physician must submit supporting clinical information and seek authorization, typically from a third-party company, before the imaging study can be performed. For example, one academic neuroradiology section participated in a radiology utilization management program and found that approximately 20% of studies were not performed, including inappropriate use of lumbar spine MR imaging for uncomplicated low back pain, saving approximately $150,000 in

unnecessary imaging.[39] Another similar strategy to reduce the use of inappropriate imaging is to use computerized radiology order entry with decision support. The clinician is prompted to answer specific clinical questions to determine appropriateness of the study at the time an order is placed. For example, Virginia Mason, an integrated health care system, developed a decision support system to promote effective imaging of outpatient low back pain using institutionally derived decision rules based on primary literature, evidence-based guidelines, and collaboration with their specialty colleagues. If the study was determined to be inappropriate at the time of physician order entry, the lumbar spine MR imaging could not be ordered and the patient was offered a same-day appointment for clinical evaluation in a dedicated clinic for low back pain. Using this strategy, the rates of outpatient lumbar spine MR imaging decreased nearly 25%.[40]

Physician and patient education programs are necessary to improve the practice of evidence-based imaging. To overcome the lack of physician awareness and understanding of evidence-based imaging guidelines, medical education, particularly early in training, is necessary. Moreover, evidence-based imaging, including ACR Appropriateness Criteria, should be taught and practiced as part of radiology residency training.[41] Education programs for patients can help to address their expectations and misperceptions regarding the need for imaging while maintaining patient satisfaction.[42] For example, the ACR/Radiology Society of North America Choosing Wisely marketing campaign is aimed at reducing radiation exposure in adults by educating patients and providers on decreasing the number of unnecessary studies.[43] Educating patients regarding appropriateness of imaging as well as the costs and risks of ineffective imaging would require a cultural leap in the practice of medicine; however, this may prove more effective if patients were required to pay for ineffective imaging tests out of their own pockets.

Legislation for health care reform and tort reform are necessary to foster the practice of evidence-based imaging. Self-referral is a significant barrier to the practice of evidence-based imaging; because it is entrenched, it will continue until there is effective legislation to prohibit it. Fee-for-service compensation, which rewards overuse, could be replaced with systems that reward effective utilization such as managed care, accountable care organizations, or value-based reimbursement. Fear of litigation for practicing evidence-based imaging will need to be addressed with tort reform.

RADIOLOGISTS' ROLE IN THE FUTURE OF EVIDENCE-BASED IMAGING

Radiologists are critical to the future practice of evidence-based imaging. First, radiologists should help bridge the gaps in imaging evidence by participating in comparative-effectiveness studies. The Institute of Medicine has prioritized topics for comparative-effectiveness research, which include comparing treatment strategies for low back pain, comparing effectiveness of new versus traditional imaging technologies for neurologic indications, and comparing effectiveness of imaging by radiologists and nonradiologists.[44] Moreover, the American Recovery and Reinvestment Act of 2009 provided the Agency for Healthcare Research and Quality and the National Institutes of Health with more than $1 billion to specifically support these types of comparative-effectiveness studies.

Ultimately, expanding the role of the radiologist from image interpretation to utilization consultation is critical for promoting the practice of evidence-based imaging and can add value to an organization.[45] Radiologists are in a strong position to serve as expert consultants to guide effective, evidence-based imaging. For example, in one survey, more than 60% of clinicians would be willing to consult with a radiologist for assistance in determining the appropriate examination for a patient.[33] Radiologists have long been recognized for their expertise in interpreting studies. It is now paramount that our health care system recognizes and rewards radiologists for their expertise as consultants who can help guide effective utilization in evidence-based imaging.

REFERENCES

1. Organization for Economic Cooperation and Development. Health at a glance 2011: OECD indicators. Paris: Organization for Economic Cooperation & Development; 2012.
2. Fuchs VR, Sox HC Jr. Physicians' views of the relative importance of thirty medical innovations. Health Aff (Millwood) 2001;20(5):30–42.
3. Sawyer F. Carolina East gets new MRI equipment. Sun Journal. 2011. Available at: http://www.newbernsj.com/articles/center-102688-new-carolinaeast.html. Accessed December 20, 2011.
4. Levin DC, Rao VM, Parker L, et al. Bending the curve: the recent marked slowdown in growth of noninvasive diagnostic imaging. AJR Am J Roentgenol 2011;196(1):W25–9.
5. Medicare Payment Advisory Commission. Report to the Congress: issues in a modernized Medicare program. MedPAC; 2011. Available at: http://www.medpac.gov/documents/Jun11DataBookEntireReport.pdf. Accessed December 19, 2011.
6. Babiarz LS, Yousem DM, Parker L, et al. Utilization rates of neuroradiology across neuroscience specialties in the private office setting: who owns or leases the scanners on which studies are performed? AJNR Am J Neuroradiol 2012;33(1):43–8.
7. Lehnert BE, Bree RL. Analysis of appropriateness of outpatient CT and MRI referred from primary care clinics at an academic medical center: how critical is the need for improved decision support? J Am Coll Radiol 2010;7:192–7.
8. Pham HH, Landon BE, Reschovsky JD, et al. Rapidity and modality of imaging for acute low back pain in elderly patients. Arch Intern Med 2009;169(10):972–81.
9. Angrisano C, Farrell D, Kocher B, et al. Accounting for the cost of health care in the United States. Washington, DC: McKinsey Global Institute; 2007.
10. Berrington de Gonzalez A, Mahesh M, Kim K-P, et al. Projected cancer risks from computed tomographic scans performed in the United States in 2007. Arch Intern Med 2009;169(22):2071–7.
11. Martin BI, Deyo RA, Mirza SK, et al. Expenditures and health status among adults with back and neck problems. JAMA 2008;299(6):656–64.
12. Medina LS, Blackmore CC. Evidence-based imaging: optimizing imaging in patient care. 1st edition. New York: Springer; 2005.
13. Jarvik JG, Hollingworth W, Martin B, et al. Rapid magnetic resonance imaging vs radiographs for patients with low back pain: a randomized controlled trial. JAMA 2003;289(21):2810–8.
14. Gilbert FJ, Grant AM, Gillan MG, et al. Low back pain: influence of early MR imaging or CT on treatment and outcome–multicenter randomized trial. Radiology 2004;231(2):343–51.
15. Hollingworth W, Jarvik JG. Technology assessment in radiology: putting the evidence in evidence-based radiology. Radiology 2007;244(1):31–8.
16. Fryback DG, Thornbury JR. The efficacy of diagnostic imaging. Med Decis Making 1991;11(2):88–94.
17. Jarvik JJ, Hollingworth W, Heagerty P, et al. The Longitudinal Assessment of Imaging and Disability of the Back (LAIDBack) study: baseline data. Spine 2001;26(10):1158–66.
18. Lurie JD, Birkmeyer NJ, Weinstein JN. Rates of advanced spinal imaging and spine surgery. Spine 2003;28(6):616–20.
19. Pengel LH, Herbert RD, Maher CG, et al. Acute low back pain: systematic review of its prognosis. BMJ 2003;327(7410):323.
20. Ash LM, Modic MT, Obuchowski NA, et al. Effects of diagnostic information, per se, on patient outcomes in acute radiculopathy and low back pain. AJNR Am J Neuroradiol 2008;29(6):1098–103.

21. Chou R, Fu R, Carrino JA, et al. Imaging strategies for low-back pain: systematic review and meta-analysis. Lancet 2009;373(9662):463–72.

22. Davis PC, Wippold FJ 2nd, Brunberg JA, et al. ACR appropriateness criteria on low back pain. J Am Coll Radiol 2009;6(6):401–7.

23. American College of Radiology. ACR Appropriateness Criteria® overview. Available at: http://www.acr.org/SecondaryMainMenuCategories/quality_safety/app_criteria/overview.aspx. Accessed December 10, 2011.

24. Chou R, Qaseem A, Snow V, et al. Diagnosis and treatment of low back pain: a joint clinical practice guideline from the American College of Physicians and the American Pain Society. Ann Intern Med 2007;147(7):478–91.

25. Agency for Health Care Policy and Research. Acute low back problems in adults: assessment and treatment. Agency for Health Care Policy and Research. Clin Pract Guidel Quick Ref Guide Clin 1994;(14):iii–iiv, 1–25.

26. Williams CM, Maher CG, Hancock MJ, et al. Low back pain and best practice care: a survey of general practice physicians. Arch Intern Med 2010;170(3):271–7.

27. Carman KL, Maurer M, Yegian JM, et al. Evidence that consumers are skeptical about evidence-based health care. Health Aff (Millwood) 2010;29(7):1400–6.

28. Schers H, Wensing M, Huijsmans Z, et al. Implementation barriers for general practice guidelines on low back pain a qualitative study. Spine 2001;26(15):E348–53.

29. Verbeek J, Sengers MJ, Riemens L, et al. Patient expectations of treatment for back pain: a systematic review of qualitative and quantitative studies. Spine 2004;29(20):2309–18.

30. Wilson IB, Dukes K, Greenfield S, et al. Patients' role in the use of radiology testing for common office practice complaints. Arch Intern Med 2001;161(2):256–63.

31. Shye D, Freeborn DK, Romeo J, et al. Understanding physicians' imaging test use in low back pain care: the role of focus groups. Int J Qual Health Care 1998;10(2):83–91.

32. Baker R, Lecouturier J, Bond S. Explaining variation in GP referral rates for x-rays for back pain. Implement Sci 2006;1:15.

33. Bautista AB, Burgos A, Nickel BJ, et al. Do clinicians use the American College of Radiology appropriateness criteria in the management of their patients? AJR Am J Roentgenol 2009;192(6):1581–5.

34. Dagenais S, Tricco AC, Haldeman S. Synthesis of recommendations for the assessment and management of low back pain from recent clinical practice guidelines. Spine J 2010;10(6):514–29.

35. Levin DC, Rao VM, Kaye A. Turf wars in radiology: recent actions against self-referral by state governments, commercial payers, and Medicare—hope is on the horizon. J Am Coll Radiol 2008;5(9):972–7.

36. Hillman BJ, Joseph CA, Mabry MR, et al. Frequency and costs of diagnostic imaging in office practice—a comparison of self-referring and radiologist-referring physicians. N Engl J Med 1990;323(23):1604–8.

37. Mello MM, Chandra A, Gawande AA, et al. National costs of the medical liability system. Health Aff (Millwood) 2010;29(9):1569–77.

38. Berlin L. Errors of omission. AJR Am J Roentgenol 2005;185(6):1416–21.

39. Friedman DP, Smith NS, Bree RL, et al. Experience of an academic neuroradiology division participating in a utilization management program. J Am Coll Radiol 2009;6:119–24.

40. Blackmore CC, Mecklenburg RS, Kaplan GS. Effectiveness of clinical decision support in controlling inappropriate imaging. J Am Coll Radiol 2011;8(1):19–25.

41. Mainiero M. Incorporating ACR practice guidelines, technical standards, and appropriateness criteria into resident education. J Am Coll Radiol 2004;1:277–9.

42. Deyo RA, Diehl AK, Rosenthal M. Reducing roentgenography use. Can patient expectations be altered? Arch Intern Med 1987;147(1):141–5.

43. Anon. Radiation safety in adult medical imaging—image wisely. Available at: http://www.imagewisely.org/. Accessed December 20, 2011.

44. Institute of Medicine. Initial national priorities for comparative effectiveness research. Washington, DC: National Academies Press; 2009.

45. Allen B, Levin DC, Brant-Zawadzki M, et al. ACR white paper: strategies for radiologists in the era of health care reform and accountable care organizations: a report from the ACR Future Trends Committee. J Am Coll Radiol 2011;8:309–17.

Radiology Reporting and Communications: A Look Forward

Adam E. Flanders, MD*, Paras Lakhani, MD

KEYWORDS

• Radiology reporting • Communication • Medical error • Structured reporting

KEY POINTS

- The content and prose method of radiology reporting has remained essentially unchanged for more than 100 years.
- The radiology report is a multifunctional document that provides information at a number of levels: it provides essential details about the provided service and can be an invaluable reference in the billing process.
- Physician-to-physician communication errors are frequently cited as one of the most common causes of medical errors and it is one of the top five indications for medical malpractice in radiology. The most frequent communication error is failure of the radiologist to directly contact the referring physician.
- The possibilities for reintroducing structured reporting into the clinical setting have much greater promise because of improvements in technology, developments in infrastructure and the general requirement to extract more information from the reports generated.
- Doing more with less has become the objective throughout all of medicine and the real goal is to improve the quality of the "product" using less time and resources.

REPORTING IS COMMUNICATION

In very generic terms, radiology provides two essential services: imaging studies and reports. The centerpiece of a radiologist's communication is the radiology report. It is an encapsulation of a consultation including the question posed, the clinical information provided at the time of service, the type of imaging test performed, a detailed recounting of the imaging findings, and a summary or impression that ties the relevance of the findings to the clinical problem and a communication. The report is also a medicolegal document: it codifies the type of service provided, the clinical query the service is attempting to answer, the success or limitations of the provided service, the findings identified, and the conclusions derived based on the findings.[1,2] In addition to its clinical function, the report can be used for billing, accreditation,

quality improvement, research, and teaching, and can serve as a means to communicate with the patient.[2]

Although there have been phenomenal technologic advances in the generation and transmission of the written word through digital dictation and the Internet, the content and format of radiology reporting has changed very little since the first medical radiograph was produced. In most instances, a radiology report is prose text that capitulates a list of imaging findings with a summation that addresses these findings in the context of a given clinical problem. For many years, radiology reports were handwritten documents. Carbon paper allowed for generation of multiple copies of the handwritten report at the time the study was interpreted such that a copy of the report could be included in the patients' film records and in the patient chart. Delivery of reports (and

Department of Radiology, Thomas Jefferson University Hospital, Suite 1080B Main Building, 132 South Tenth Street, Philadelphia, PA 19107, USA
* Corresponding author.
E-mail address: adam.flanders@jefferson.edu

Neuroimag Clin N Am 22 (2012) 477–496
doi:10.1016/j.nic.2012.04.009

films) to referring physicians used conventional courier methods that sometimes took days or weeks to arrive. The advent of the analog dictation system allowed radiologists to focus more of their attention on the images (rather than the report) by simultaneously speaking while studying the actual images. The adaptation of this technology helped to increase throughput and improved the overall appearance of the transcriptionist typed report. Additional technologies, such as the ubiquitous facsimile machine and copy machine, adopted into clinical practices improved the dissemination of information, speed of delivery, and consistency of the delivered product. Speech recognition (SR) technology has enabled real-time transcription of radiology reports, and Internet technologies now provide instantaneous communication and delivery of reports and critical findings. Although the layout of radiology reports has changed little since the profession began, the changing structure and governance of medicine suggest that radiology reporting requires a makeover.

Although tremendous strides have been made in the technology used to generate and disseminate the radiology report, the content and prose method of reporting has remained essentially unchanged for more than 100 years. It is still the primary method of communication between radiologist and clinician. The report can be created and delivered more efficiently, yet the message it contains still varies considerably in style and clarity. One of the earliest observers of the vagaries of radiology reporting was a nineteenth century radiologist named Preston Hickey who also served as one of the first editors of the *American Journal of Roentgenology*.[3] Hickey was a proponent of proper radiology reporting skills and he advocated for the need of a standardized approach to radiograph reporting as early as 1899.[4] He introduced the term "radiograph" as a substitute for roentgenogram, and he was the first to describe the process of radiographic "interpretation," which he defined as creating a differential diagnosis from radiographic findings that might lead to a conclusion based on probabilities similar to a pathologic report.[5] Even at that time when the specialty was in its infancy, Hickey observed that the styles of reporting of the day were so ambiguous such that it was impossible to formulate a diagnosis or even relate the findings to the clinical problem. Hickey was a strong advocate for the use of a standardized report (similar to pathology) and urged the consistent use of standardized nomenclature in reporting.[4,6] He was particularly disappointed by the general lack of requirements to teach trainees the skills to describe and characterize abnormalities.[3] His

devotion to this concept led to his recommendation that candidacy for membership to the American Roentgen Ray Society be predicated on review of 100 example reports submitted with a candidate's application. A candidate's membership could be denied based on the quality of their reports.[3] A contemporary of Hickey, Charles Enfield, wrote of the importance of conveying meaning to the reported findings and the essential need to express opinion or conclusion as to the significance of the findings.[7]

The insights of Hickey and Enfield into the value of the quality of radiology reports are no less relevant today than they were a century ago. These individuals recognized that the added value of the radiologist was in his or her skill to assemble a cogent, concise, and unambiguous description of relevant findings that addressed the given clinical problem. This required a careful choice of terminology, good organization, and brevity whenever possible.[2] A critical component of the report was the synthesis of the findings to formulate a conclusion or summary that takes into account the clinical status of the patient and the unanswered question being addressed in the report.

WHAT ARE THE FEATURES OF A COMPLETE RADIOLOGY REPORT?

Developing a comprehensive understanding of effective reporting and communication is predicated on having a broad understanding of who uses the report and how they use it. Radiology now serves many "customers" including the patient.[1] The radiology report is a multifunctional document that provides information at several levels: it provides essential details about the provided service and it can be an invaluable reference in the billing process. As radiologists, we think of the report as documentation of the presence, absence, progression, or remission of a disease or the description of a therapeutic procedure. There is no single "consumer" of the radiology report: users include the ordering provider; other specialists; trainees and health professionals; and other radiologists (who may refer to the report at a later time or interpret additional modalities). In the modern era of the personalized health record, the patient has also become an important consumer of medical reports.[1] Primary care physicians are dependent on the content of the radiology report, whereas specialists (eg, neurosurgeons, neurologists, or orthopedic surgeons) depend on review of the imaging studies themselves and use the report as a reference. Clinicians have less time to review radiology reports, particular ones that are overly wordy or complex. The radiologist needs to be cognizant that in many instances only a portion of the report (typically the impression or summary) is actually read; therefore, particular care must be taken in crafting the summary or conclusion of any report.[8] As face-to-face contact between referring physicians and radiologists has waned with dissemination of enterprise imaging distribution systems, the quality of the written report has taken on even greater importance and the obligation to improve the product is more relevant today than it was in the past.[9]

A well-crafted report should be structured to maximize value to the consumer of that information. In most cases that is the ordering physician. However, attitudes among radiologists as to what constitutes a quality report are variable. All reports have three cardinal features: (1) content, (2) structure, and (3) style. Compromises in any of these features can produce substantial changes to the quality of the report and can have detrimental effects on communication with the clinician and customer satisfaction. Clinician surveys of radiology report quality are often cited as justification for a fresh approach to report generation, although many of these studies suffer from bias inherent to the limited characteristics polled in each survey.[6] One of these surveys examined the relationship between report complexity and perceived report clarity by clinicians. A software program was used to objectively rate a report for inherent grammatical complexity in a collection of more than 10,000 thousand reports and then to compare whether these indices related to perceived clarity and comprehension of the report by clinicians.[10] Not surprisingly, the authors found that the indices were higher for more intricate studies. Readability indices varied by radiologist for similar studies likely reflecting stylistic and linguistic differences. Interestingly, complex reports with higher indices (ie, long, complex sentences) were perceived as less clear by the clinicians and conveyed less diagnostic certainty than shorter and more concise reports. The authors suggested that complex reports may be perceived as unreliable or associated with obfuscation and that elements of uncertainty should be expressed directly.[11,12]

Several published editorial and opinion pages are devoted to the appropriate structure and style of the radiology report.[4,6–8,10,12–16] Much of what has been established for correct reporting is based on preference surveys from clinicians.[9,17] Although there is a general lack of evidence regarding effectiveness of reporting guidelines and much of what has been written is based on anecdote and opinion, one can conclude that a report should follow a logical structure and reach a conclusion similar to a scientific paper or abstract (Box 1).[6] A proper report is accurate, concise, clear, and pertinent in style.[16] Clinicians also have a preference for structured reports over pure unstructured free-text report.[9,18] The American College of Radiology (ACR) handbook for residents recommends that the prototypical radiology report be divided into six main sections: (1) examination, (2) history and indication, (3) technique, (4) comparison, (5) findings, and (6) impression.[19] It has been suggested that a good radiology report allows the referring physician to generate a mental picture of the abnormalities identified; it suggests a probability of specific diagnosis and the next appropriate steps for management.[16] Therefore, it is imperative that the report should always be geared to address the needs of the referring clinician.[6] It should clearly describe the study or procedure, the pertinent findings, a differential diagnosis ranked by order of likelihood, and recommendations for additional evaluation if indicated. The report should address any specific question (eg, "no demyelinating lesions" in an instance where "rule out demyelinating disease" is specified).[6,8]

Reporting style is important because if used incorrectly it can adversely affect the clarity of the report. For this reason, a report should not be overly technical or wordy. Coakley and colleagues[16] recommend adhering to three main stylistic guidelines of (1) brevity, (2) clarity, and (3) pertinence. Armas[20] advocated the six-Cs of correct radiology reporting: (1) clarity, (2) correctness, (3) confidence, (4) concision, (5) completeness, and (6) consistency (Box 2). There are numerous editorials and opinion papers on best practices for radiology reporting offer stylistic "do's and don't's" for crafting good dictation style (Box 3, Table 1). Two additional nonstylistic ("C") qualities were proposed by Reiner and

---

Box 1
General radiology report layout and format structure

Title of examination

Relevant clinical history or indication

Technique

Use of comparisons

Findings

Conclusion/summary/impression

Data from Wallis A, McCoubrie P. The radiology report: are we getting the message across? Clin Radiol 2011;66(11):1015–22.

Box 2
Eight ideal "C" qualities of the radiology report

Clarity

Correctness

Confidence

Concision

Completeness

Consistency

Communication

Consultation

Data from Reiner BI, Knight N, Siegel EL. Radiology reporting, past, present, and future: the radiologist's perspective. J Am Coll Radiol 2007;4(5):313–9; and Armas RR. Qualities of a good radiology report. AJR Am J Roentgenol 1998;170(4):1110.

Box 3
Examples of "hedge" vocabulary to indirectly express uncertainty

- Density or opacity
- Apparent
- Appears
- Possible/possibly
- Borderline
- Doubtful/uncertain/unlikely
- Suspected
- Indeterminate
- Identified
- Seen
- No definite/gross/obvious/overt/evidence of
- No significant (eg, lymphadenopathy)
- Possible
- Probable
- Suggested
- Suspected
- Suspicious
- Vague
- Clinical correlation needed
- If clinically indicated
- Equivocal
- May represent
- Worrisome or concerning for...

Data from Wallis A, McCoubrie P. The radiology report: are we getting the message across? Clin Radiol 2011;66(11):1015–22.

colleagues[11] (communication and consultation), both of which have become the mantra for radiology quality and safety.

A critical quality of effective radiology reporting today is "timeliness." An interpretation that is delivered after a critical management decision has been made has no inherent value.[21] In this modern healthcare era of cost containment, with emphasis on reductions in length of stay with concurrent improvements in quality and safety, staying competitive and relevant mandates that radiology must deliver a quality product in a time frame that maximizes impact on patient care.[11] Technology has had the largest positive impact in expediting report delivery with the advent of SR, integrated picture archive and communications systems (PACS), radiology information systems (RIS), speech solutions, and dissemination of electronic medical records.

Report timeliness has been augmented with the advent of SR technology. Although not as ubiquitous as soft copy PACS, there has been continued and steady growth of SR installations in practices of all sizes. The advantages include rapid generation of a nicely formatted product, immediate verification of the content, near instantaneous delivery by facsimile machine or e-mail, and virtual elimination of transcription costs. The principle disadvantages of SR include requisite typing skills, frequent SR errors, and the loss of radiologist efficiency inherent to self-correction of these errors.[22] The frequency of SR errors is not insignificant. One study that assessed errors in breast imaging reports found that SR error rates were typically eight times the rate higher than conventional transcription, independent of experience or academic rank.[23]

Although there are a myriad of quality measures in any radiology practice, two metrics that are heavily scrutinized are report turnaround time (period between examination completion and finalized dictation) and report quality. Although report turnaround is perhaps easier to measure, report quality has no defined metrics associated with it. As such, report quality is frequently tied to error rates. Radiologic errors are often divided into observational (perceptual) and cognitive (interpretative). Errors in radiology reporting are not uncommon with estimates averaging around 30% overall but with a range of 26% to 90% in some series.[24] Lehr and colleagues[25] found that errors rates were similar across modalities and that there was no relationship between frequency of errors and radiologist experience or time spent interpreting radiographs. Reducing medicolegal risk can be accomplished by addressing reporting error rates.

Table 1
Text or phrases to avoid in the radiology report

Selected Guidelines	Example	
	Before	After
Avoid beginning strings of sentences with "There is…" or "There are…"	"*There is* a lacunar infarction in the left basal ganglia. *There is* mass effect on the third ventricle. *There is* a punctate focus of hemorrhage"	"Lacunar infarction in left basal ganglia with an internal microhemorrhage and mass effect on the third ventricle"
Limit differential diagnoses to four or less	"Differential diagnosis includes multiple sclerosis, infection, demyelination, inflammation, metastases, microvascular disease and headaches"	"Diagnosis favors a demyelinating process"
Avoid "clinical correlation is suggested" or "if clinically indicated"; offer a useful suggestion whenever possible	"New area of lucency in the right pons for which clinical correlation is advised"	"New lucency in the right pons; diffusion MR imaging is recommended to assess for acute infarction"
Avoid redundant words	"Again redemonstrated is the small protrusion of disk material on the right at C5/6 resulting in a mild degree of compression and deformation of the ventral spinal cord without signal changes"	"Unchanged right central C5/6 disk herniation with cord deformation"
Avoid abbreviations	GBM PCOM Mets	Glioblastoma multiforme Posterior communicating artery Metastases
Use "normal" or "unremarkable"	"No acute abnormality is seen"	"Normal brain"
Avoid the use of first person	"I don't see any hemorrhage"	"No hemorrhage"
Avoid the use of "was not seen on the prior study…"	"Enhancing mass in the right frontal lobe was not seen on the prior study but is unchanged in size"	"Enhancing mass in the right frontal lobe is unchanged in size compared with prior study"
Use the phrase "evidence of" for observations that can only be inferred and not observed directly	There is no evidence of hemorrhage or hydrocephalus (brain CT)	There is no evidence of demyelinating disease (brain CT)
Avoid the phrase "cannot be excluded"	"5-cm irregularly enhancing mass in the right temporal lobe; a glioblastoma is to be excluded"	"5-cm irregularly enhancing mass in the right temporal lobe is most likely a glioblastoma"

Adapted from Kahn CE Jr, Langlotz CP, Burnside ES, et al. Toward best practices in radiology reporting. Radiology 2009;252(3):852–6.

Although perceptual errors can be reduced through additional training or double-readings, the cause of interpretive errors can be multifactorial and not necessarily directly tied to inadequate knowledge. Lack of access to appropriate prior studies or reports and relevant clinical information may also inadvertently contribute to reporting errors. These factors can be addressed with some of the newer technologic solutions that augment integration of relevant clinical information to the radiologists' desktop at the time of interpretation.[26]

COMPONENTS OF THE REPORT

The basic elements of a radiology report have been described at length in the ACR's Practice

Guideline for Communication.[2,27,28] This should include patient identifying information, imaging procedure descriptions, clinical indications, imaging findings, and summary information (Table 2). Additional elements potentially include key images; multimedia (sound and video); and documentation of critical communications (eg, person notified, level of criticality, date and time of notification).[2]

A concise statement of the relevant clinical history is an often-overlooked, but important component of the complete radiology report. The accuracy of the contents of this section cannot be overstated because it conveys to the reader what the radiologist understood to be the clinical problem posed at the time of delivery of service. If no information has been provided then this needs to be clearly stated in the report and can be tied into the level of diagnostic uncertainty in the impression or conclusions section.[14] Subcomponents of the history section should include

a statement of the patient's underlying condition; the indication (or justification) for the study; and what relevant prior studies were used in the evaluation (when applicable) (see Table 2). SR technology integrated with RIS offers some time savings by passing examination-specific RIS field values to prepopulate header information in each report, such as patient demographics, study performed, date and time of service, and any free-text entries from the ordering physician or registrar regarding history or clinical indication. Reliance on this prepopulated data has proved to be problematic. Studies have shown that the validity of this preentered historical information is frequently inaccurate, incomplete, irrelevant, or erroneous. In one reported audit of CT requests comparing the consistency of electronic data entry with handwritten prescriptions the authors found that 49% of free-text electronic entries were either incomplete or discordant with paper requests. Half of the incomplete histories were deemed clinically

Table 2
Components of the standard radiology report

Report Section	Content
Administrative information	Imaging facility Referring provider Date and time of service
Patient identification	Name Identifier (medical record number of equivalent) Date of birth Sex
Clinical history	Medical history Risk factors Allergies, if relevant Reason for examination, including medical necessity
Imaging technique	Time of image acquisition Imaging device Image acquisition parameters, such as device settings; patient positioning; and interventions (eg, Valsalva maneuver) Contrast materials and other medications administered (including name, dose, route, and time of administration) Radiation dose
Comparison	Date and type of previous examinations reviewed, if applicable
Observations (findings)	Narrative description or itemization of findings, including measurements, image annotations, and identification of key images
Summary (impression or conclusion)	Key observations, inferences, and conclusions, including any recommendations
Communication	Verbal communication of critical and important findings including date and time and identity of recipient
Signature	The date and time of electronic signature for each responsible provider, including attestation statement for physicians supervising trainees if applicable

Adapted from Kahn CE Jr, Langlotz CP, Burnside ES, et al. Toward best practices in radiology reporting. Radiology 2009;252(3):852–6; with permission.

significant and 69% of disagreements between electronic entry and paper were also considered clinically significant.[29] The convenience of having this important part of the report "predictated" has made radiologists less aware of the need to always verify the relevance of the information before it is automatically propagated to their reports. Some radiologists even hold to the fallacy that the information that has been prepopulated into a report from another information system must remain unaltered even if that information is determined to be erroneous or irrelevant. To the contrary, this section of the report should encapsulate the entire clinical context of the radiologic examination known at the time of delivery of service; if different or supplemental clinical information is made available at the time of interpretation then this should be corrected and recorded in the report.

The technique section of the report (see **Table 2**) should elaborate on specifics of the study beyond the modality and examination type, which are part of the chargemaster like procedure name and billing codes (eg, MR brain with and without contrast). Contrast dosage (when applicable) is compulsory. In general, the technique section should specify just enough supplemental information about the examination that another radiologist will understand whether there were any inherent limitations as to how the data were acquired; recapitulating the procedure name (eg, MR imaging of the brain with contrast was performed) is insufficient. Examples might include review of scanning planes, field strength of the scanner in the case of MR imaging, and reconstructions or pulse sequences that were part of the imaging data reviewed at the time of interpretation. Exhaustive technical detail is not appropriate; just enough information to be able to reconstruct what was done. If an intervention is being reported (eg, myelogram, angiogram, or spine procedure) then a detailed accounting of all steps performed from consultation and consent, complications, and condition of the patient at the conclusion of the procedure is mandatory. This is also an important area to specify any possible technical limitations that might constrain diagnostic quality or create uncertainty.

The findings or observations section (see **Table 2**) is generally the longest portion of the report. Construction of this section organized by organ, disease process, or other structure is the basis of a standardized or structured report (**Table 3**). If a nonitemized format is used then the description of findings should be in decreasing order of importance or significance and present tense should always be used.[12] Consistent and unambiguous terminology is the most important recommendation

when describing the actual imaging findings.[13] Findings should be graded in terms of severity using reproducible modifiers, such as mild, moderate, or severe, although criteria remain highly subjective unless this is based on a uniform and validated standard vocabulary, such as the Nomenclature for Degenerative Disc Disease in the Lumbar Spine.[15,30] When measurements or other quantitative values are stated, one should adhere to best practices, such as the North American Symptomatic Carotid Endarterectomy Trial for carotid stenosis[31] or Response Evaluation Criteria in Solid Tumors[32] to assess tumor response. Use of negation is valuable only when detailing results that are pertinent to the clinical question or indication. Incidental findings should be cited judiciously and in rank order of importance.[16]

The impression, summary, or conclusion of the report should be formulated carefully because it may be the only portion of the report that the referring physician actually reads.[8] First and foremost, the impression should always address the clinical question or indication; this demonstrates that the radiologist understood the primary clinical problem.[6] A well-crafted conclusion should synthesize the meaning or significance of the findings in the context of the clinical situation; it should not merely recapitulate the findings section. If the observations consist of "solitary, centrally necrotic focus of T2 hyperintensity measuring 6 cm in diameter in the right frontal lobe," do not repeat "solitary, centrally necrotic focus of T2 hyperintensity measuring 6 cm in diameter in the right frontal lobe" in the impression when "primary glial tumor in the right frontal lobe" is a more appropriate conclusion. Differential diagnoses are helpful provided that they are not comprehensive and exhaustive and are welcomed by most physicians. Because recommendations for additional imaging (when appropriate) and nonimaging investigations were overwhelmingly preferred by general practitioners this information should also be included in the "impression" (see **Tables 2** and **3**),[17] or within a separate "recommendations" subsection within the report.

COMMUNICATIONS

The requirements of the 2005 National Patient Safety Goal of the Joint Commission on Accreditation of Healthcare Organizations for the improvement of the effectiveness of communication among caregivers has mandated the practice and documentation of timely and efficient critical results reporting.[33] Physician-to-physician communication errors are frequently cited as one of the most common causes of medical errors and

Table 3
Structured MR brain reporting template from the Radiological Society of North America's reporting template library

Clinical history	• Medical history • Risk factors • Allergies, if relevant • Reason for examination, including medical necessity: [headache | stroke | dizziness | trauma]
Imaging technique	• Time of image acquisition • Imaging device: MRI • Image acquisition parameters, such as device settings, patient positioning, interventions (eg, Valsalva maneuver) • Contrast materials and other medications administered (including name, dose, route, and time of administration) • Radiation dose
Comparison	• Date and type of previous examinations reviewed, if applicable
Observations	• Extra axial spaces: [normal in size and morphology for the patient's age* | widened] • Hemorrhage: [none*; subdural; subarachnoid; epidural, intraventricular, parenchymal] • Ventricular system: [normal in size and morphology for the patient's age* | enlarged | small] • Basal cisterns: [normal* | enlarged | small] • Cerebral parenchyma: [normal*; microvascular changes; infarction; encephalomalacia; gliosis; hemorrhage] • Midline shift: [none* | leftward shift | rightward shift] • Cerebellum: [normal*] • Brainstem: [normal*]
Other	• Calvarium: [normal*; nondepressed fracture; depressed fracture; osteolysis; sclerosis] • Vascular system: [normal* | vascular calcifications (CT) | appropriate arterial and dural sinus flow voids (MR imaging)] • Visualized paranasal sinuses: [clear* | scattered mild inflammatory mucosal thickening] • Visualized orbits: [normal*] • Visualized upper cervical spine: [normal*] • Sella and skull base: [normal* | partially empty sella | left/right mastoid air cell fluid]
Summary (or impression)	• An itemized list of key observations, including any recommendations

From Flanders AE. RSNA Radiology Reporting Templates: MR brain. Available at: http://www.radreport.org/template/0000045. Copyright (c) 2009, Radiological Society of North America, Inc. (RSNA); used with permission.

it is one of the top five indications for medical malpractice in radiology.[2,26,34,35] The most frequent communication error is failure of the radiologist to directly contact the referring physician.[34] There are tremendous misperceptions about what constitutes a "critical" or "urgent" value that warrants a direct communication and what the radiologist's true obligation is in conveying this information; one neuroradiologist may only initiate a call on discovery of a stroke or unexpected hemorrhage, whereas another may alert the clinician to the presence of an unexpected mucous retention cyst. That being said, the Joint Commission requires radiology practices to maintain an established a list of critical results and have policies to communicate such, but leaves it up to the institutions to determine what types of results are considered critical.[33]

Although reports remain the centerpiece for communication with clinical colleagues, it is not the sole means of communication and face-to-face or verbal contact is mandated in several circumstances. The ACR standard for communication specifies that the radiologist is responsible for directly contacting the referring physician (or their designate) about "urgent, clinically significant or unexpected findings." These include: (1) findings that require immediate or urgent intervention (eg, new cerebral hemorrhage or infarction); (2) findings that are discordant with the prior interpretation of the same imaging study (a prior examination or a preliminary report of the current examination) where failure to act may affect the patient's health (eg, tumefactive multiple sclerosis lesion previously interpreted as a primary brain tumor); and (3) unexpected findings that may be seriously adverse to the patient's health (eg, renal mass discovered on a lumbar spine CT) (Box 4).[27] Direct (verbal) communication is mandated in these circumstances and proof or documentation (audits) of regular communication is expected by regulatory agencies, such as the Joint Commission.[33]

Of the more than 160 guidelines created by the ACR none has been as contentious or as hotly debated as the ACR Communications Guideline.[28,36] It has been heralded as a practice standard for more than a decade, yet there has been considerable debate about the actual value (or harm) the Guideline poses to radiologists. Some argue that the guidelines, although well intended, are out of date given the now contemporaneous report generation made possible by SR and secure digital delivery of reports. Others contend that communication requirements have been only partly mitigated against by improvements in interpretation and report turnaround time and that these technologic breakthroughs have even compounded the problem by increasing the expectations by referring physicians.[26] Other factors that have increased the burden of communications overall include the growing dependency on complex imaging studies for routine clinical management (eg, routine trauma screening with MR imaging) with the concomitant increase in overall workload; the proliferation of PACS; and enterprise image delivery solutions, which have had the detrimental impact of decreasing routine interaction with clinicians.[26] Some even contend that ACR Guidelines have been responsible for encouraging litigation for communication-related errors. However, case law has shown that radiologists were being held subject to liability long before the Guidelines existed.[35]

Because communication methods are varied and complex, acknowledgment and documentation of communication transactions is often problematic and inconsistent. Radiologists are often misinformed as to where their obligation to communicate important findings begins and ends. The ACR specifies "that non-routine communications be handled in a manner most likely to reach the attention of the treating or referring physician in time to provide the most benefit to the patient."[27] Ideally, the radiologist should personally deliver important findings to the physician of record or the physician who ordered the examination. The time commitment for responsible communication is not insignificant. With increasing workloads and other demands on their time, radiologists find it more challenging to divert their attention from interpretation to brokering telephone calls. One estimate is that it takes an average of 5 minutes to verbally report an examination, which equates to approximately 1000 radiologist man-hours annually.[36]

Identifying the most responsible caregiver at any given moment can also present a challenge. This is notable in teaching facilities where "teams" of physicians may change daily or by shift. The conveyed information is not a "hot potato" that can be simply passed on to any other person

---

Box 4
Situations that may require nonroutine communication initiated by the radiologist

- *Findings that suggest a need for immediate or urgent intervention*:

  ○ Generally, these cases may occur in the emergency and surgical departments or critical care units and may include pneumothorax, pneumoperitoneum, or a significantly misplaced line or tube.

- *Findings that are discrepant with a preceding interpretation of the same examination and where failure to act may adversely affect patient health*:

  ○ These cases may occur when the final interpretation is discrepant with a preliminary report or when significant discrepancies are encountered upon subsequent review of a study after a final report has been submitted.

- *Findings that the interpreting physician reasonably believes may be seriously adverse to the patient's health and are unexpected by the treating or referring physician*:

  ○ These cases may not require immediate attention but, if not acted on, may worsen over time and possibly result in an adverse patient outcome.

Adapted from American College of Radiology (ACR). ACR practice guidelines for communication of diagnostic imaging findings. [online publication]. Reston (VA): American College of Radiology (ACR); 2010.

and then dismissed by the radiologist. The radiologist should attempt to deliver the information to a person who in the radiologist's judgment is best suited to act on that information; a verbal report to a clerk or secretary is no substitute for the ordering physician or housestaff directly caring for the patient. For many of these reasons, the hand-off of the information is not always ideal.

A related concept that is difficult to assess but is as important as the information being conveyed is the perception of acknowledgment. The individual accepting responsibility for the verbal report must be able to acknowledge that they comprehend the information being conveyed and the level of urgency for acting on the information. There must be some assurance from the receiving party that they are capable of intervening directly on behalf of the patient or that they will be able to urgently relay this information to a direct caregiver on the clinical team. This can be difficult to assess in a 60-second telephone call and when doubts arise it may oblige the radiologist to search for a more appropriate surrogate.[35] The ACR recommends doctor-to-doctor communications but recognizes that there are circumstances when a suitable surrogate is allowable when the primary physician is not available. Ultimately, if the radiologist is unable to locate an appropriate responsible provider (off hours interpretation or in the instance of self or third-party referrals) then the interpreting radiologist may need to deliver the findings directly to the patient with advice for next appropriate steps (eg, emergency room visit).[27,35]

The final step in the communications cycle is complete documentation of the actual communication. This should include the date and time of communication in addition to the exact identity and role of the party who received and acknowledged this information. In the event of litigation, good documentation serves as strong evidence that a radiologist acted reasonably. However, the absence of documentation implies or leaves open doubt that the communication never took place.[35] The ACR communications task force also recommends documentation of all consultations in the medical record or within the radiology report (if possible) but otherwise in an alternate location. Even "curbside" consultations of outside studies should be preserved with some form of documentation and the completeness of the material provided at the time the opinion was rendered (eg, if the study was submitted with insufficient history, clinical information, prior reports, or examinations). The documentation should include the relevant clinical question, information available at the time of review, and any technical limitations of the study.[35]

Even through best efforts, documentation of critical results reporting is often incomplete or absent largely because of the manual processes that are involved and lack of integrated information technology solutions. Similarly, means for auditing critical results reporting frequency can be primitive even with current technologies, although data mining algorithms have proved that this process can be automated.[37] Closing the communications loop has become one of the fundamental challenges of radiology practices. Although there are some commercial technologic solutions available that can help augment the process, there are no complete turnkey solutions that can easily coordinate all communication activities.

Many radiology practices have found it cost and time effective to hand off communications responsibilities to a call center or secretary whose sole responsibility is to broker and record communications between the interpreting radiologists in the reading room and clinical staff. There are also commercial informatics capabilities that can augment portions of the entire communications cycle, although fully integrated solutions that verify receipt of messages are yet to be realized. A system that closes the entire communications loop without a radiologist's intervention is unrealistic and problematic to implement. An ideal solution might incorporate a real-time natural language processor that monitors dictations in-progress for use of critical values (eg, new hemorrhage, infarction, or cord compression) that could alert the interpreting radiologist by offering to initiate a critical result communication. Once the radiologist acknowledged the need to contact a physician, the system would work behind the scenes to aggregate the identities and communication preferences of the most appropriate providers based on a set of rules. This requires interrogation of multiple information systems depending on the complexity of the clinical entity. Direct paging, text paging, and voice messaging would be instantiated behind the scenes by the system while the radiologist continues to work. The returned telephone call and caller identity would be saved in a voice file and the verbal information transaction would then be appended automatically to the report. Unreturned pages or voice mails could initiate a call to another person on the clinical team after a given period of time. For less urgent findings, such as an incidental lung nodule seen on a CT of the cervical spine, an email or text-messaging notification system to alert the referring provider may be acceptable and preferred; in such a case, an appropriate reply from the provider could acknowledge of receipt of the findings. Ultimately, if all automated methods for communication were unsuccessful, an alert could be provided back to the requesting radiologist or clerk to manage the process manually. Logs of all transactions could be used for quality assurance and regulatory reporting. Closure of the entire communications loop with referring physicians should also include noncritical but important follow-up, such as recommendations for additional studies. Unfortunately, all of these steps are time-consuming and most radiologists are reluctant or unenthusiastic about having to append previously dictated reports to document communication.

STRUCTURED REPORTING

The mention of structured or standardized reporting sometimes invokes fear and trepidation in the minds of many radiologists. Those that are old enough to remember the first implementations of structured reporting systems recall an overly engineered device with touchscreens and awkward complicated dropdown menus taking the place of the familiar microphone and prose dictation. Individuality in dictation style was lost in favor of a rigid, tightly constrained, and unbending structure that was built around menus of multiple-choice answers. Most loathsome was the real concern that adoption of any structured reporting technology maximizes radiologist inefficiency and reduces accuracy by diverting the radiologist's attention to the report instead of the images.[21] Some of these concerns were true; most of the point-and-click implementations developed nearly a decade ago were found to be inefficient, rigid, and limited in scope. Today, however, the possibilities for reintroducing structured reporting into the clinical setting has much greater promise because of improvements in technology, developments in infrastructure, and the general requirement to extract more information from the reports generated.

A standardized report or itemized report incorporates a regular and predictable organization to a report without imposing a controlled vocabulary. The familiar report template used in speech systems today is a form of a standardized report and is easily implemented on modern SR systems (Fig. 1, see Table 2).[21] The template imposes a general arrangement to the report with machine or manually enterable fields, such as patient demographics, examination description, technique, contrast, indication, findings, and impression. Key field elements may be specified, such as ventricles, extra-axial spaces, and parenchyma, with placeholders for free-text entry. There are no constraints of a controlled terminology

in a standardized report. Note that the organizational elements and subheadings in the itemized report (see Fig. 1; Fig. 2) make the report easier to read and understand than the unstructured free-text report (Fig. 3). Numerous surveys have shown that clinicians prefer standardized or itemized reporting compared with free-form prose reports.[3,9,21,22] Naik and colleagues[22] found a strong preference for computer-generated itemized reports by referring clinicians and radiologists. Preferences notwithstanding, another study reported no productivity advantages for either the radiologist creating the report or the referring provider who reads the report.[18] In contrast, a brain MR imaging cohort study that compared structured reporting with conventional free-text dictation showed no significant difference in report accuracy or completeness.[38] Although there are many advantages in using a consistent report structure to improve readability and comprehension, there are potential deficiencies.

A structured report, by contrast, is organized into logical sections and uses standardized terminology.[2,21,39] It has three principle characteristics. First, the format is organized and divisible by paragraphs and headings that contain the basic headings of the report similar to a standardized report (eg, impression, technique, findings). Second, the subheadings of the report are organized in a consistent (and logical) fashion labeled by key anatomic elements (eg, marrow elements, intervertebral disk spaces, spinal cord). The third key attribute of a structured report is the use of standard language.[21] This is the characteristic component of the structured report and its implementation prompts the most concern by radiologists because it forces the radiologist to adhere to a very specific terminology. An example of a structured brain MR imaging report template is shown in Table 3. Report examples of unstructured prose text, an itemized or standard report, and a pure structured report are shown in Figs. 1–3. Note that although the information in the free-text unstructured report (see Fig. 3), the standardized or itemized report (see Fig. 1), and the structured report using controlled terminology (see Fig. 2) is essentially identical, the structured format is less ambiguous, more comprehensible, and consumed more efficiently.

It has been shown that reports that use non-standard language are less comprehensible that reports that adhere to standardized lexicons.[21,40] A report built on standardized terminology can be more easily abstracted into data elements that can support research, quality improvement initiatives, and teaching. The clear advantage of structured reports is that the information is

Name: Joe BagO'Donuts
MRNUM: 12345678
DOB: 02/14/1930
Ordering provider: Dr. Bilbo Baggins' MD PhD
Exam: MRI Brain with Contrast.
Date of Service: 01/01/2000 22:53
History/Indication: Uncontrolled hypertension. Patient reports visual blurriness for last several months.

Technique: MR study of the brain and brainstem consists of multiple sagittal, axial and coronal images using T1, T2, gradient echo and DWI pulse sequences. The T2 weighted images are limited by motion artifact.

Contrast: 15 cc of intravenous Gadovist were administered into the right forearm without reaction.

Comparison: Current exam is evaluated in comparison to a prior MRI study of the brain dated 10/11/1999 and a CT from Man's Best Hospital dated 07/04/1999.

Findings: There is a new area of cortical encephalomalacia with subcortical gliosis in the right occipital pole which was not present on either of the prior studies representing interval development of a cortical infarction. There is no corresponding DWI abnormality.

There is no intra- or extra-axial hemorrhage. No midline shift or mass effect is present. The ventricular system is normal in size and configuration for age. There are discrete and confluent changes in the central and subcortical white matter attributed to microvascular disease.

The visualized paranasal sinuses are clear.

Incidental finding of a bone island in the left frontal bone.

Impression: Age-indeterminate right occipital cortical infarction with stable underlying microvascular changes.

Fig. 1. Standardized report of a brain MR image using consistent section headings and prose or free-text dictation.

recorded in a manner such that it is more amenable to data retrieval and reuse.[21] Tools built to analyze data from a structured report can be leveraged as the basis for decision support tools used during interpretation with comparison with relevant prior imaging studies. Data easily extracted from a structured report can serve as the cornerstone for developing business analytics including documentation of service, report turnaround, billing, throughput and efficiency evaluations, quality assurance, and regulatory compliance measures.[2] Similarly, structured reporting may facilitate data-mining efforts for retrospective research purposes. A structured format lends itself to enhancing critical results reporting

and potentially can capture receipt and acknowledgment of critical imaging findings by the referring physician. The structured report could also contain a comprehensive list of data elements that record all patient interactions with technologists, nurses, and trainees.[2]

If structured reporting offers the best possible communication solution with the highest accuracy and the capability to extract data for other purposes, why then has it not proliferated in step with SR technology and template or itemized reporting? The answer is threefold: (1) the absence of a useable standardized lexicon for radiology, (2) shortage of vetted and validated reporting templates, and (3) the lack of an attractive

Name: Joe BagO'Donuts
MRNUM: 12345678
DOB: 02/14/1930
Ordering provider: Dr. Bilbo Baggins' MD PhD
Exam: MRI Brain with Contrast.
Date of Service: 01/01/2000 22:53
Performing technologist: Ann Coulter, RT
History/Indication: Uncontrolled hypertension. Patient reports visual blurriness for last several months.

Technique:
- **Field strength**: 1.5T
- **Vendor**: Philips Integra
- **Planes**: Sagittal, axial and coronal
- **Pulse sequences**: T1, T2, GRE, DWI
- **Quality**: Diagnostic

Contrast:
- Type: Gadovist
- Volume:
- Route: IV, left hand.

Comparison:
- 10/11/1999 11:31 - MRI brain
- 07/04/1999 23:45 - CT brain (Man's Best Hospital).

Findings:
- **Extra axial spaces:** normal in size and morphology for the patient's age
- **Hemorrhage:** None
- **Ventricular system:** Normal in size and morphology for the patient's age
- **Basal cisterns:** Normal.
- **Cerebral parenchyma:**
    - New encephalomalacia and gliosis right occipital pole.
    - Generalized microvascular changes subcortical regions.
- **Midline shift:** None.
- **Cerebellum:** Normal.
- **Brainstem:** Normal.

Other:
- **Calvarium**: Normal
- **Vascular system:** Appropriate arterial and dural sinus flow voids.
- **Visualized Paranasal sinuses:** Clear.
- **Visualized Orbits:** Normal.
- **Visualized upper cervical spine:** Normal.
- **Sella and skull base:** Normal.

Impression: Age-indeterminate right occipital cortical infarction with stable underlying microvascular changes.

Fig. 2. Structured report of a brain MR image using itemized anatomic lists and controlled vocabulary.

technology to create structured reports. Historically, input systems for structured reporting have been labor intensive requiring substantially greater keyboard input, mouse clicks, and interaction with hierarchical menus and a protracted learning curve. The additional diversion imposed by heavy interaction with the reporting software may have an untoward effect on eye dwell time because the radiologist is forced to spend less time searching the image for abnormalities in exchange for increased attention to report generation.[21] The primary concern in adopting a pure structured reporting solution is a loss of radiologist accuracy and efficiency.

To address one of the prime deficiencies in adoption of standardized reporting and to identify

Name: Joe BagO'Donuts
MRNUM: 12345678
DOB: 02/14/1930
Ordering provider: Dr. Bilbo Baggins' MD PhD
Exam: MRI Brain with Contrast.
Date of Service: 01/01/2000 22:53
History/Indication: Uncontrolled hypertension. Patient reports visual blurriness for last several months.

Comment: An MRI of the brain was performed with and without Gadolinium. The paranasal sinuses that are seen on this study show no significant sinus disease. There is no gross evidence of hemorrhage seen. There is no midline shift or mass effect seen. The ventricles are pretty much normal except the third ventricle seems kind of big. There is a density in the left frontal bone. There are bright spots in the white matter near the surface of the brain on the T2 weighted images which could be due to multiple sclerosis, UBOs, infections, inflammations, stroke and possibly tumors. There is no evidence of abnormal enhancement that is seen. I feel that this most likely represents ischemic disease but clinical correlation is suggested. These findings were likely present on the prior studies. There is also some volume loss in the right occipital area which I believe is secondary to trauma. Clinical correlation is recommended.

Impression: There are hyperintensities in the brain white matter for which clinical correlation is advised.

Fig. 3. Prose, free-text dictation of a brain MR image with minimal structure and no controlled terminology.

and promote best practices the Radiological Society of North America (RSNA) established a Radiology Reporting Committee in 2008.[41] The committee, consisting of radiology subspecialists and informatics experts, developed a strategy for creation of standardized report templates by domain experts and a means to incorporate these templates into commercial speech systems. Input was also provided by colleagues from cardiology, gastroenterology, surgical pathology, and oncology who have established structured reporting practices in their own specialties. The committee endorsed the data element requirements of the ACR Communications Guidelines[27] and suggested supplemental requirements that would include multimedia (sound and video), key images, and data elements for critical results reporting including person notified, level of criticality, and date and time of notification.[2] Additional requirements suggested by the committee included data elements that would facilitate decision support, data mining, quality improvement initiatives, and regulatory compliance.[2] The group also emphasized the need to tailor the presentation of reports to the individual reader, such as patients, specialists, general practitioners, and radiologists, by emphasizing or deemphasizing specific data elements. It is important to recognize that the goal of the RSNA Reporting Committee is not to define the content or format of any specific report. The committee's charge has been to develop infrastructure that helps to identify and promote best practices for using reporting templates that have been developed by various subspecialty societies, individual institutions, or practices. A technologic framework was developed by the committee based on open standards (nonproprietary) architectures such that the exchange of templates could be easily accomplished between disparate or competing products. This required adoption of several web technologies, such as extensible markup language, which has a natural compatibility with industry standards, such as the Health Level 7 Clinical Document Architecture and the Digital Imaging and Communications in Medicine Structured Reporting protocols.[2] A radiology reporting template browser (http://www.radreport.org/) is available to help search, view, and download contributed templates based on subspecialty, organ system, or modality. Twenty neuroradiology templates are available on the site (http://www.radreport.org/specialty/nr) for examination or to download into one's favorite SR system. A sample MR imaging brain template from the RSNA is shown in **Table 3**. The committee plans to allow users to submit their own templates to the Web site, provide feedback, and rate existing templates in a fashion similar to commercial Web sites, such as Amazon.com. It is hoped that this will foster increased participation and improve the quality of the templates.

The most famed example of success of structured reporting in radiology is the Breast Imaging Reporting and Data System (BI-RADS) for mammography reports. Mandated by the Food and Drug Administration more than 20 years ago, BI-RADS has unified reporting of breast cancer to such a degree that it has radically changed the importance of mammography in diagnosis of breast disease. Standardization has reduced variability in reporting and improved the clarity of communications between radiologist and referring physician.[9,21,42] It has provided benchmarks for many outcome variables that are now required of practices for quality assurance and performance. Moreover, because all practices now evaluate the disease in the same fashion, BI-RADS provides a framework for data collection and auditing.[42] Think of the possibilities if the same could be done for human astrocytomas, multiple sclerosis, degenerative disk disease, and stroke.

Structured reporting relies on the consistent use of standardized or controlled terminologies to reduce ambiguity and to provide concise definitions or concepts in reports. The concept of imposing standardized terminology in radiology report generation is not new; Preston Hickey and other likeminded contemporaries of his day were insistent that this guideline was most important in maintaining quality communication with clinicians.[4] Although it took more than 80 years for organized radiology to devise a radiology-specific set of controlled terminology, it is finally available through the radiology lexicon (RadLex).[43] The need for a standard lexicon is straightforward: although radiologists worldwide are trained to perform dictation, they all have their own idiosyncratic word preferences that may be related to differences in style, training, and age. Terms with identical or similar meaning may have different implications to the consumer of that information. There are a myriad of examples, such as "disk protrusion," "herniation," or "focal bulge"; "multifocal bright spots," "unidentified bright object," or "ovoid-shaped hyperintense lesion"; and "infarct," "stroke," "cerebral ischemia," or "infarction." Not only does use of consistent terminology improve the fidelity of the message to the reader, but it also enhances the capability for machine learning of the same information. This opens numerous possibilities for expanding the function of the radiology report for such applications as quality assurance, decision support, and business analytics.

Indexes of radiology terms have been around for a long time for manual reference. The RSNA maintained a bound index of terms for its portfolio of educational products including the annual meeting. The ACR created an innovative reference known as the "ACR Index" for cataloging radiology teaching files that paired anatomic and pathologic codes for easy retrieval. As material moved online, these manual indexes revealed important shortcomings. Implementation of computer databases allowed for storage of an unlimited number of terms and their interrelationships to other terms. The Systemized Nomenclature of Medicine–Clinical Terms (SNOMED–CT) originally created by the American College of Pathologists contains more than 350,000 concepts used in electronic medical records. Others commonly in use include the National Library of Medicine's Unified Medical Language System (UMLS) and Medical Subject Headings, Logical Observation Identifiers Names and Codes (LOINC) sponsored by the Regenstrief Institute, and the Foundational Model of Anatomy (FMA) developed by the University of Washington School of Medicine. The FMA is an example of ontology. Ontologies differ from dictionaries or lists of terminologies in an important aspect: they map the relationships between terms. Terms are organized into classes with attributes that determine if it is a "part of" another term and what class the term belongs to (eg, anatomy, pathology). Although dictionaries compile their content in alphabetical order regardless of their meaning, ontologies organize terms based on their relationship to one another in what is known as an "inheritance hierarchy" or "taxonomy." An additional feature supported by ontologies is the ability to build interrelationships to similar terms (eg, synonyms or synonymy) either within a single index or between multiple, independent indexes. These capabilities foster the creation of machine-based intelligence or inference; a computer using the appropriate ontologic model could potentially "understand" the relationships of the terms in a radiology report.

RadLex is a RSNA-sponsored project. Multiple domain experts from all subspecialties in radiology and in associated clinical subspecialties helped to collect, verify, and organize the terminology, which captures specific terms in general use by radiologists that are not otherwise represented in other libraries, such as SNOMED, UMLS, or LOINC. The first version was launched in 2006 with more than 30,000 terms. Some of the terms are modality specific, such as hyperintense, radiolucent, hypoechoic, ground-glass, and so forth.

The progenitor of RadLex and success story for adoption of structured reporting in clinical practice has been the BI-RADS project.

Despite the proliferation of public taxonomies and controlled terminologies in medicine, there were no medical terminology systems available to meet the needs of online radiology indexing.[43,44] To address this limitation the RSNA initiated the RadLex project, whose primary goal is to identify and fill these gaps in current public medical terminology systems.[43] RadLex is designed to be the single exemplar source of terminology in medical imaging. The lexicon provides a uniform structure for indexing terms from a variety of sources including radiology teaching files, radiology reports, and research data.[21] In addition to supplementing radiology-specific anatomic and pathologic terms, RadLex also addresses terms related to perceptual and anatomic difficulty (eg, uncertainty), diagnostic quality of images, devices, procedures, and imaging techniques.[43] Terms that are in common use by radiologists but are not found in any lexicon (eg, hyperintense, susceptibility, hypoechoic) are codified in RadLex. RadLex now contains more than 34,000 unique terms. Each is identified by a unique code that can be connected to related terms, such as synonyms, acronyms, and variants of terms.[2] RadLex is a "living document"; it is continuously supplemented and updated and it has been linked with many of the popular terminologies, such as SNOMED-CT and BrainInfo (http://braininfo.rprc.washington.edu).

There are substantial external pressures that mandate greater standardization and accountability in health care, much of which is driven by the desire for more evidence-based decisions and cost containment. Metrics tied to improved efficiency, pay-for-performance, quality assurance, risk management, and meaningful use of health information technology are all ultimately standards-based and are how we will be judged now and in the future. Although one of radiology's strengths as a specialty has been in its development and adoption of new technologies, it has been slow to catch on to structured reporting. Other specialties, such as cardiology and gastroenterology, have already successfully implemented structured reporting into their workflow and have tied it to reimbursement and pay-for-performance activities. Some have suggested that structured reporting is more manageable and less complex in these other specialties than in radiology, where the number of organ systems and disease process are cross cutting across all specialties.[1,39,45]

Those who are under the misapprehension that these kinds of initiatives do not or will not apply to them must recognize that the federal government already has developed pay-for-performance type programs that tie financial incentives (or penalties) to compliance with specific activities. One program sponsored by the Centers for Medicare and Medicaid Services that is specifically tied to a quality measure as it relates to radiology reporting is the Physicians Quality Reporting System (PQRS) (formerly known as the Physician Quality Reporting Initiative). The PQRS is a voluntary reporting program that provides incentive payment to physicians and eligible professionals who can provide data that satisfactorily reflect compliance with specific quality measures in radiology claims data.[46] There are specific measures for diagnostic and interventional radiology and nuclear medicine and radiation oncology. Moreover, measures number 10, 145, and 195 are specific to neuroradiology (Box 5). To qualify for these incentive payments, a practice must be able to accurately document a percentage or proportion of reports that includes the dictation requirement specified. A standardized or structured report template that already includes the requisite terminology is easier to deploy and implement than requiring each radiologist to remember to include the language in every report. The most important concept to recognize is that pay-for-performance and PQRS are just the beginnings of government intervention into payment and penalties related to radiology services. Some of the newest and toughest challenges on the horizon are related to proving "meaningful use" of health information technology in one's practice and meeting the benchmarks and key performance indicators that are just being developed by the federal government.[47] Many of the requirements for radiologists will be crafted in the next year and the dates to meet compliance are in 2015 and 2016. Many of the metrics that radiologists will be held accountable for in these new regulations will be based on the clarity of information in their radiology reports. Success or failure depends on how well they prepare for it.

CHALLENGES

Many of the changes in the healthcare environment present new challenges to radiology. Reiner and colleagues[11] subdivide these challenges into four areas: (1) improve quality and reduce errors, (2) reduce medicolegal risk and improve clinical outcomes, (3) increase productivity and workflow, and (4) increase profitability. Doing more with less has become the objective throughout all of medicine and the real goal is to improve the quality of the "product" using less time and resources. We

---

Box 5
Neuroradiology-specific reporting requirements for PQRS incentives

- #10 Stroke and stroke rehabilitation: CT or MR imaging reports
  - ○ Percentage of final reports for CT or MR imaging studies of the brain performed within 24 hours of arrival to the hospital for patients aged 18 years and older with either a diagnosis of ischemic stroke or transient ischemic attack or intracranial hemorrhage or at least one documented symptom consistent with ischemic stroke or transient ischemic attack or intracranial hemorrhage that includes documentation of the presence or absence of each of the following: hemorrhage, mass lesion, and acute infarction.
  - ○ Dictation requirement: include the following statement in the findings section: "There is (or is no) acute infarction, hemorrhage, or mass lesion."
- #145 Radiology: exposure time reported for procedures using fluoroscopy
  - ○ Percentage of final reports for procedures using fluoroscopy that include documentation of radiation exposure or exposure time.
  - ○ Dictation requirement: include the following statement in the technique section: "The total fluoroscopy exposure time was ____ minutes."
- #195: Stenosis measurement in carotid imaging reports
  - ○ Percentage of final reports for all patients, regardless of age, for carotid imaging studies (neck MR angiography, neck CT angiography, neck duplex ultrasound, carotid angiography) performed that include direct or indirect reference to measurements of distal internal carotid diameter as the denominator for stenosis measurement.
  - ○ Dictation requirement: include the following statement in the technique section: "All qualitative and quantitative assessments of carotid bifurcation and proximal internal carotid artery stenoses are made referencing the distal internal carotid artery."

---

are at a technical crossroads, whereby routine standardized and structured reporting of imaging studies could facilitate multiple simultaneous functions. A report based on structured data using controlled terminology is powerful and versatile. The metadata (visible and hidden) in the report can be structured and presented in an unlimited array of formats. Moreover, the metadata can be accurately linked to other data repositories to provide greater depth or "meaning" to the report (Fig. 4). Entering the report would be based on an efficient combination of interactions with the PACS and prose dictation entered into an "intelligent" adjudicated master template containing essential key data elements relevant to that disease (eg, presence of hemorrhage, type of hemorrhage, intra-axial or extra-axial process, solid vs cystic, and so forth). The modality (eg, MR imaging), examination type or procedure (eg, proton MR spectroscopy), and the protocol used (eg, single voxel PRESS, with TE of 144 milliseconds) would automatically populate specific fields in the report as would relevant clinical history that matches International Classification of Diseases-9 (or -10) codes. These data would help facilitate billing and departmental business metrics. The raw data elements could be used to automatically generate multiple kinds of documents useful to

different consumers based on their needs. For example, a prose text report could be machine generated from the structured data elements entered by the radiologist. Ambiguous and stylistic language that is commonly used to express uncertainty could be essentially eliminated. Instead, uncertainty of a finding could be qualified with a discrete modifier. Because structured and controlled terminology is better "understood" by machines, critical results reporting could be initiated automatically just by the discovery of the use of specific key values in the report.[37] Moreover, multiple kinds of reports could be created using different structure or style depending on a clinician's preference or background. Because reports need to satisfy different consumers, one approach is for the radiologist to provide a complete report cataloging all the findings. In this way, with advances in computer technology, different consumers could then call on specialized "views" of that report tailored for their specialized needs. Such technology could be available in the foreseeable future. Even now, many referring physicians look at specific headings or subheadings of reports to find pertinent information for their clinical needs (eg, a spine surgeon looking at the musculoskeletal section of the report looking for potential disk herniations). Because

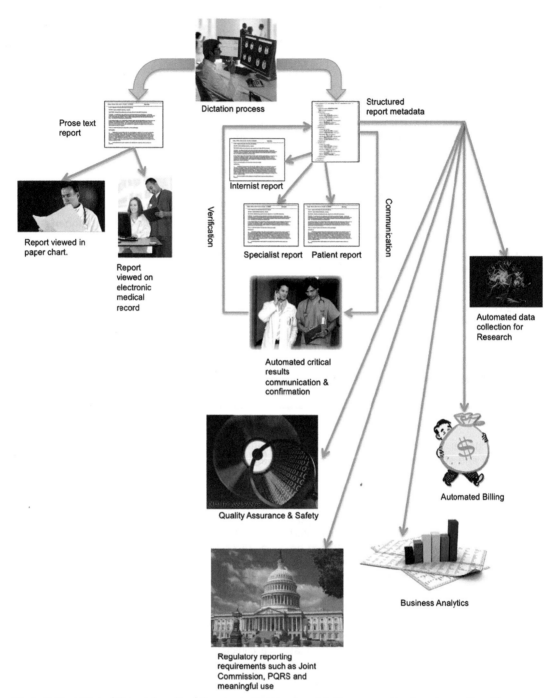

Prose text report

Dictation process

Structured report metadata

Report viewed in paper chart.

Report viewed on electronic medical record

Internist report

Verification

Specialist report   Patient report

Communication

Automated critical results communication & confirmation

Automated data collection for Research

Quality Assurance & Safety

Automated Billing

Regulatory reporting requirements such as Joint Commission, PQRS and meaningful use

Business Analytics

Fig. 4. Comparison of the work cycle of the conventional prose dictation versus structured reporting. The conventional report (*left*) is consumed in print or in the electronic health record and filed. The rich metadata in the structured report (*right*) is capable of spawning multiple automated processes including versions of reports, communication of critical results with verification, automated data collection for research, business analytics, quality assurance, regulatory requirements, and billing.

standardized terminology is used in the template, ontologic relationships to related terms are inherent to the system. This would allow for report creation of varied complexity ranging from a patient-centric report (using laypersons terminology) to a report that fully incorporates higher-level terminology for a specialist (eg, Macdonald criteria for multiple sclerosis for a neurologist).

Because controlled terminologies are used to generate the report, ontologic relationships can be used to link to relevant reference materials at the appropriate level for the reader. The unformatted metadata for each report could be sent to national registries, such as the ACR, to help monitor and benchmark regional, local, and national use and monitor radiation dose. This would help departments and institutions automatically monitor and meet quality assurance requirements mandated by the Joint Commission and other regulatory bodies. The report metadata in some instances may trigger a reminder from pathology to provide the radiologist with feedback on the histopathology of the brain biopsy based on the recent brain MR image that he or she recently interpreted. Areas of deficiency in knowledge could trigger delivery of customized continuing educational learning modules to help each individual radiologist improve their own knowledge gaps and benchmark performance against peers in the academic and private practice environment. All of this is possible with an evolution in the product: the radiology report.

REFERENCES

1. Dunnick NR, Langlotz CP. The radiology report of the future: a summary of the 2007 Intersociety Conference. J Am Coll Radiol 2008;5(5):626–9.
2. Kahn CE Jr, Langlotz CP, Burnside ES, et al. Toward best practices in radiology reporting. Radiology 2009;252(3):852–6.
3. Gagliardi RA. The evolution of the X-ray report. AJR Am J Roentgenol 1995;164(2):501–2.
4. Hickey P. Standardisation of roentgen-ray reports. AJR Am J Roentgenol 1922;9:422.
5. Hickey P. The interpretation of radiographs. J Mich Med Soc 1904;3:496.
6. Wallis A, McCoubrie P. The radiology report: are we getting the message across? Clin Radiol 2011; 66(11):1015–22.
7. Enfield C. The scope of the roentgenologist's report. JAMA 1923;80:999.
8. Clinger NJ, Hunter TB, Hillman BJ. Radiology reporting: attitudes of referring physicians. Radiology 1988;169(3):825–6.
9. Schwartz LH, Panicek DM, Berk AR, et al. Improving communication of diagnostic radiology findings through structured reporting. Radiology 2011;260(1): 174–81.
10. Sierra AE, Bisesi MA, Rosenbaum TL, et al. Readability of the radiologic report. Invest Radiol 1992; 27(3):236–9.
11. Reiner BI, Knight N, Siegel EL. Radiology reporting, past, present, and future: the radiologist's perspective. J Am Coll Radiol 2007;4(5):313–9.
12. Hall FM. Language of the radiology report: primer for residents and wayward radiologists. AJR Am J Roentgenol 2000;175(5):1239–42.
13. Friedman PJ. Radiologic reporting: the hierarchy of terms. AJR Am J Roentgenol 1983;140(2):402–3.
14. Hall FM. Clinical history, radiographic reporting, and defensive radiologic practice. Radiology 1989; 170(2):575–6.
15. McLoughlin RF, So CB, Gray RR, et al. Radiology reports: how much descriptive detail is enough? AJR Am J Roentgenol 1995;165(4):803–6.
16. Coakley FV, Liberman L, Panicek DM. Style guidelines for radiology reporting: a manner of speaking. AJR Am J Roentgenol 2003;180(2):327–8.
17. Grieve FM, Plumb AA, Khan SH. Radiology reporting: a general practitioner's perspective. Br J Radiol 2010;83(985):17–22.
18. Sistrom CL, Honeyman-Buck J. Free text versus structured format: information transfer efficiency of radiology reports. AJR Am J Roentgenol 2005; 185(3):804–12.
19. Getting started: a guide to year one of radiology residency ACR resident and fellow section [Internet], 2009. Available at: http://rfs.acr.org/pdf/ GettingStarted_Handbook.pdf. Accessed February 11, 2012.
20. Armas RR. Qualities of a good radiology report. AJR Am J Roentgenol 1998;170(4):1110.
21. Weiss DL, Langlotz CP. Structured reporting: patient care enhancement or productivity nightmare? Radiology 2008;249(3):739–47.
22. Naik SS, Hanbidge A, Wilson SR. Radiology reports: examining radiologist and clinician preferences regarding style and content. AJR Am J Roentgenol 2001;176(3):591–8.
23. Basma S, Lord B, Jacks LM, et al. Error rates in breast imaging reports: comparison of automatic speech recognition and dictation transcription. AJR Am J Roentgenol 2011;197(4):923–7.
24. Berlin L. Reporting the "missed" radiologic diagnosis: medicolegal and ethical considerations. Radiology 1994;192(1):183–7.
25. Lehr JL, Lodwick GS, Farrell C, et al. Direct measurement of the effect of film miniaturization on diagnostic accuracy. Radiology 1976;118(2):257–63.
26. Siegel EL. Goodbye, Mr. Cox: time for automated closure of the radiology communication loop. Appl Radiol 2005;34:312.
27. ACR practice guidelines for communication of diagnostic imaging findings. Reston, Virginia: American College of Radiology; 2010.
28. Lucey LL, Kushner DC, American College of Radiology. The ACR guideline on communication: to be or not to be, that is the question. J Am Coll Radiol 2010;7(2):109–14.
29. Agarwal R, Bleshman MH, Langlotz CP. Comparison of two methods to transmit clinical history

information from referring providers to radiologists. J Am Coll Radiol 2009;6(11):795–9.

30. Fardon DF, Milette PC. Combined Task Forces of the North American Spine Society, American Society of Spine Radiology, and American Society of Neuroradiology. Nomenclature and classification of lumbar disc pathology. Recommendations of the combined task forces of the North American Spine Society, American Society of Spine Radiology, and American Society of Neuroradiology. Spine (Phila Pa 1976) 2001;26(5):E93–113.

31. Clinical alert: benefit of carotid endarterectomy for patients with high-grade stenosis of the internal carotid artery. National Institute of Neurological Disorders and Stroke and Trauma Division. North American Symptomatic Carotid Endarterectomy Trial (NASCET) investigators. Stroke 1991;22(6):816–7.

32. Sasaki T. New guidelines to evaluate the response to treatment "RECIST." Gan To Kagaku Ryoho 2000;27(14):2179–84.

33. Joint Commission on Accreditation of Healthcare Organizations. 2005 hospital national patient safety goals. Goal: improve the effectiveness of communication among caregivers. Oakbrook terrace (IL): Joint Commission on Accreditation of Healthcare Organizations; 2004.

34. Physician Insurers Association of America and American College of Radiology. Practice standards claims survey. Rockville (MD): Physician Insurers Association of America; 1997.

35. Kushner DC, Lucey LL, American College of Radiology. Diagnostic radiology reporting and communication: the ACR guideline. J Am Coll Radiol 2005;2(1):15–21.

36. Brantley SD, Brantley RD. Reporting significant unexpected findings: the emergence of information technology solutions. J Am Coll Radiol 2005;2(4):304–7.

37. Lakhani P, Langlotz CP. Automated detection of radiology reports that document non-routine communication of critical or significant results. J Digit Imaging 2010;23(6):647–57.

38. Johnson AJ, Chen MY, Swan JS, et al. Cohort study of structured reporting compared with conventional dictation. Radiology 2009;253(1):74–80.

39. Sistrom CL, Langlotz CP. A framework for improving radiology reporting. J Am Coll Radiol 2005;2(2):159–67.

40. Khorasani R, Bates DW, Teeger S, et al. Is terminology used effectively to convey diagnostic certainty in radiology reports? Acad Radiol 2003;10(6):685–8.

41. RSNA informatics reporting. Radiology reporting initiative [Internet].; 2009; cited January 15 2012. Available at: http://www.rsna.org/informatics/radreports.cfm. Accessed February 11, 2012.

42. Langlotz CP. ACR BI-RADS for breast imaging communication: a roadmap for the rest of radiology. J Am Coll Radiol 2009;6(12):861–3.

43. Langlotz CP. RadLex: a new method for indexing online educational materials. Radiographics 2006;26(6):1595–7.

44. Langlotz CP, Caldwell SA. The completeness of existing lexicons for representing radiology report information. J Digit Imaging 2002;15(Suppl 1):201–5.

45. Langlotz CP. Structured radiology reporting: are we there yet? Radiology 2009;253(1):23–5.

46. CMS physicians quality reporting system (PQRS) [Internet]: American College of Radiology; 2011; cited January 15, 2012. Available at: http://www.acr.org/SecondaryMainMenuCategories/quality_safety/p4p/FeaturedCategories/P4PInitiatives/pqri.aspx. Accessed February 11, 2012.

47. Flanders AE. The real "meaning" behind meaningful use. Radiographics 2010;30(5):1329–33.

Combating Overutilization
Radiology Benefits Managers Versus Order Entry Decision Support

David M. Yousem, MD, MBA

KEYWORDS

• Overutilization • Radiology benefits manager • Order entry decision support • Health care costs

KEY POINTS

- Radiology benefits managers (RBMs) and computerized decision support offer different advantages and disadvantages in the efforts to provide appropriate use of radiology resources.
- RBMs are effective in their hard-stop ability to reject inappropriate studies, incur a significant cost, and interpose an intermediary between patient and physician.
- Decision support is a more friendly educational product, but has not been implemented for all clinical indications and its efficacy remains unproved.

INTRODUCTION

The question of what to do about the escalating costs of providing health care to the citizens of the United States has dominated the politics of this country over the past 3 years. Although Oba-maCare versus RomneyCare versus MediCare versus MediScare are concepts that have led to divisions between conservative and liberal and libertarian and Tea Party advocates, one of the basic tenets of the debate has been that there is excess in the system. With respect to imaging, as opposed to (or perhaps in addition to) Big PHARMA, the assumption is that overutilization is a major driver in the escalation of health care expenses. This presumption emphasizes that this overutilization relates to the more expensive, higher relative value unit (RVU) procedures rather than more economical modalities. Therefore the combination of a drive from less expensive tests to more expensive tests and the overall increase in imaging tests per patient leads to the double-digit increases in imaging costs annually in the United States.[1,2] To address these issues, the insertion of an intermediary between the ordering physician and the imaging procedure has led to the 2 solutions addressed in this article: radiology benefits managers (RBMs) and physician order entry decision support (OEDS).

Before addressing the solutions, it is useful to assess the problem in greater detail because the concept of overutilization has many facets that may or may not be addressed by RBMs and OEDS. Radiologists have long held that the increased imaging costs are not borne by traditional diagnostic imaging by radiologists. The rate of escalation of imaging costs has been driven to a large extent by specialty imaging not performed by radiologists but by cardiologists and oncologists and other subspecialists.[3,4] Although this may reflect the increased incidence of cardiovascular disease and cancer in the population, the aging of the population and longer life spans, or the demand from the public for maximal health care from birth to death, radiologists often publicly opine that the increased usage is rooted in vested self-interest in a fee-for-service world. Radiologists cry "Self-referral!" (Box 1).

By self-referral, the radiology community suggests that clinicians who order tests performed by those

Russell H. Morgan Department of Radiology and Radiological Sciences, The Johns Hopkins Medical Institution, 600 North Wolfe Street, Phipps B100F, Baltimore, MD 21287, USA
E-mail address: dyousem1@jhu.edu

Neuroimag Clin N Am 22 (2012) 497–509
doi:10.1016/j.nic.2012.05.013
1052-5149/12/$ – see front matter © 2012 Elsevier Inc. All rights reserved.

<table>
<tr><td>

Box 1
Purported causes of overutilization of imaging

1. Fascination with new technologies
2. Duplication of studies from site to site
3. Inappropriate examination ordered/wrong body part imaged
4. Defensive medicine
5. Self-referral financial incentive
6. Patient demand for test
7. Studies ordered by protocol without individual consideration
8. Fraudulent activity

</td></tr>
</table>

same clinicians are acting irresponsibly and with economic motivations other than the interest of the patient. Whether a cardiologist or orthopedic surgeon has a greater tendency to order a cardiac nuclear scintigram or magnetic resonance (MR) imaging of the knee when that clinician either owns the machine and charges the technical fee or interprets the same study and charges the professional fee has been studied in the literature based largely on Center for Medicare Services (CMS) and other provider sources of data.[3–13] Most of the literature shows an ever-increasing proportion of imaging studies being conducted and interpreted by nonradiologists across the modalities with the highest RVUs.[9,10,12,14–16] These articles and others show that, when scanners and imaging studies are owned and interpreted respectively by nonradiologists, the rate of growth in utilization exceeds that of the studies referred to and performed by radiologists.[15–17] The per-patient utilization rate in CMS terms has increased more among self-referring specialties than in traditional diagnostic radiology. This per-patient rate addresses the issue of increased numbers of older patients living longer and having disease, and raises issues of vested self-interest by self-referrers leading to overutilization.

Specific examples of these influences are worth citing. They include: (1) between 1998 and 2002, private office radionuclide myocardial perfusion imaging by radiologists increased by 16%, whereas the increase for cardiologists was 101%[15]; (2) between 2000 and 2005, private office neuroradiology MR imaging examinations by radiologists increased by 83%, compared with a 254% increase by nonradiologists[10]; (3) during 2001 to 2006, private office computed tomography (CT) studies by radiologists increased by 85% versus 263% for nonradiologists[17]; (4) between 2002 and 2007, positron emission tomography (PET) studies by radiologists increased by 259%

versus 737% for nonradiologists[12]; and (5) neurologists and neurosurgeons increased their private office neuroradiology MR studies by more than 200% between 1998 and 2008 (**Figs. 1** and **2**).[18] These differences document the impact of self-referral.

Another source of overutilization is duplicate studies. In a health care system in which the average period that a patient stays with a given insurance company is just 2.3 years, the likelihood that studies performed by providers supported by 1 insurer can be accessed by clinicians from a different insurance system is low. It requires an effort that the clinicians may find burdensome. It is easier just to order a new study in your own system than to retrieve images and reports from a foreign system. When the transient allegiance to an insurance provider is coupled with an ever-mobile society, there are lost studies in the system leading to duplicate imaging because the clinicians or patients are unaware of what has been previously performed. Until a universally accessible electronic patient record is created (one of the more worthy provisions of ObamaCare), the potential for repetitive imaging is high.

Inappropriate imaging may also stem from physician ignorance. With the expanded role of imaging in making diagnoses and the increased armamentarium of MR imaging, CT, MR angiography, CT angiography, nuclear medicine, and ultrasound techniques, the array of potential studies to order becomes daunting to someone not in academic centers experiencing the advances. As an example, clinical examination, ultrasound, CT, or MR imaging can be used to diagnose an

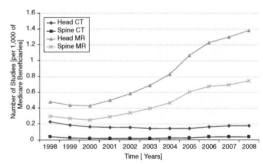

Fig. 1. Neuroradiology studies performed by neurologists in the private office setting. Use rates between 1998 and 2008 for head CT, spine CT, head MR, and spine MR for neurologist equipment owners/lessees in the private office setting. (*Adapted From* Babiarz LS, Yousem DM, Parker L, et al. Utilization rates of neuroradiology across neuroscience specialties in the private office setting: who owns or leases the scanners on which studies are performed? AJNR Am J Neuroradiol 2011;33(1):43–8; with permission.)

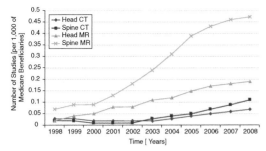

Fig. 2. Neuroradiology studies performed by neurosurgeons in the private office setting. Use rates between 1998 and 2008 for head CT, spine CT, head MR, and spine MR for neurosurgeon equipment owners/lessees in the private office setting. (*Adapted From* Babiarz LS, Yousem DM, Parker L, et al. Utilization rates of neuroradiology across neuroscience specialties in the private office setting: who owns or leases the scanners on which studies are performed? AJNR Am J Neuroradiol 2011;33(1):43–8; with permission.)

appendiceal abscess. Which should be used? What is the standard of care in 2012? Is the cost of the study a factor? Are all studies readily available in the emergency department (ED)? To keep up with the imaging guidelines in a medical system in which the radiologist is rarely used in this capacity as a consultant is daunting.

In addition, another factor that is often decried as a source for increased use is fear of litigation.[19] This input is frequently cited by physicians who blame defensive medicine as the source of many studies needed to rule out the 0% to 5% chance of an entity for fear of missing a diagnosis that may lead to a malpractice suit. The growth of imaging in the ED usually is most commonly attributed to defensive medicine because any motor vehicle collision, concussion, slip and fall, or pelvic/hip pain may harbor a subtle life-threatening lesion that is unapparent to clinical examination. The pan-scan from lower extremity to the vertex of the skull to exclude disorders in patients who are inebriated, unconscious, unreliable historians, or in accidents that have a higher rate of such injuries has led to marked imaging increases emanating from the ED. The advent of CT scanners within the ED has also led to increased use **(Table 1)**[20] and the added concern about unnecessary radiation to the populace.

Inappropriate selection of examinations was studied by Lehnert and Bree.[21] Reviewing 459 examinations performed, the investigators found that 26% were inappropriate, including examples of studies in which no tests should have been performed, the wrong test was ordered, the wrong body part was ordered, or the study was duplicative.

The rate at which a significant finding was found on these inappropriate tests was less than half the rate in those studies in which the indication and study were appropriate.

An America's Health Insurance Plans (AHIP) white paper[22] suggested several additional factors that account for inappropriate imaging, including (1) deficiencies in the quality of imaging services by those performing the test, (2) lack of information on imaging effectiveness in some clinical situations, and (3) direct-to-consumer advertising and the impact on consumer demand for these services.

It has been estimated that all of the factors discussed earlier suggest that one-third of imaging procedures are inappropriate, costing the country between $3 billion and $10 billion annually.[23]

To address several of these issues, the insertion of a pause in the system (ie, RBMs and OEDS) is a potentially worthy and cost-effective safety net. This article addresses the competitive advantages and disadvantages of each of these suggested solutions to some of the ills of our radiology procedure order and procurement system as well as suggesting future directions that may be more useful in controlling a system that has uncontrolled for too long.

RBMs

RBMs have stated goals of (1) guiding usage, (2) controlling costs, (3) guaranteeing quality, (4) smoothing patient throughput, (5) determining study appropriateness, (6) preventing redundancy, (7) improving efficiency, and (8) improving patient safety by reducing exposure to unnecessary ionizing radiation.[24] RBMs have made significant headway in the commercial insurance market and are contracted by many insurers. They are currently in operation in 50 states and control use for more than 90 million patients.[24] Medicare currently disallows the requirement for RBMs in its fee-for-service programs but not its Medicaid and Medicare Advantage plans.

The top 4 RBMS by number of patients cover about 90 million patients in the United States **(Box 2)**. They include MedSolutions (Franklin, TN), which began in 1992 and focused exclusively on so-called intelligent cost management in 1997 (www.medsolutions.com). MedSolutions was recently selected by Cigna to be its exclusive RBM for members covered in the United States. MedSolutions has worked with Cigna for 13 years, but its overall client base stands at about 25 million individuals nationwide, including Medicare Advantage beneficiaries. American Imaging Management (AIM) Inc has headquarters in Deerfield, Illinois, was

Table 1
Impact of placement of CT scanner in ED

Relationship to CT Scanner Installation	Number of Patients Seen in ED	Number of Patients Scanned with CT	% of Patients Scanned	Rate of Positive Findings (%)
Year before	48866	3884	7.9	23.3
Year after	50,611	6569	13.0	15.0
Change	1745	2685	69 (increase)[a]	35.6 (decrease)[a]

[a] Statistically significant.
Data From Oguz KK, Yousem DM, Deluca T, et al. Effect of emergency department CT on neuroimaging case volume and positive scan rates. Acad Radiol 2002;9(9):1018–24.

founded in 1989, and acquired by WellPoint Inc in 2007 (www.americanimaging.net). AIM's growth has been exceptional, from 5 million members in 2004 to 13 million in 2005, to 20 million in 2007, to 30 million in 2008, and, as of 2010, it covered 35 million members. CareCore National claims to be the largest specialty benefits manager and has bases in South Carolina and Colorado (www.carecorenational.com). Its services include cardiac imaging (established 2005), cardiac implantable devices, oncologic agents (2007), radiation therapy, pain management, and laboratory services (2008). CareCore National was founded in 1994 and currently manages services of 30 million people. National Imaging Associates (NIA) was founded in 1995, acquired by Magellan Health Services in 2006, and is headquartered in Avon, Connecticut (www.niahealthcare.com). As of 2009, NIA covered 18 million Americans.

To provide a scope of the nature of these companies, insight can be gained from the employee ranks. A company such as NIA manages approximately 400,000 studies per month. Although this is similar to the total output of a 930-bed hospital like Johns Hopkins Hospital, NIA only focuses on high-RVU studies like CT, MR imaging, cardiac nuclear medicine, and PET, and does not manage inpatient services, which are often paid for on a diagnosis-related group (DRG) system. The DRG system for inpatients yields a flat rate to the hospital based on a specific diagnosis and payment is not wholly based on use. NIA has 6000 employees, including 75 physician reviewers and 5 full-time radiologists. NIA is employed by many insurance companies to manage their imaging services. Insurance clients include Absolute Total Care, Blue Cross Blue Shield of Florida, CareSource, Cigna, Geisinger Health Plan, Highmark, Keystone Mercy Health, Magnolia Health Plan, WellPath, and Harvard Pilgrim Health Care (www.niahealthcare.com).

How does the process work? NIA reviews a physician's request for a study before its performance. Although initially this is through a computer-based system staffed by clinical service representatives (CSRs) for appropriateness, if any red flags between a (1) match of study and indications, or (2) length of symptoms (eg, MR imaging of the lumbar spine ordered within 5 days of onset of back pain with no neurologic symptoms rather than industry standard of waiting 6 weeks), or (3) recent studies are identified, a health professional (usually a nurse) intervenes. From this encounter, the requesting physician may be bumped up to a physician consultant for study approval.

General percentages suggest that 70% of studies are immediately approved based on algorithms inputted by a technical employee in the initial call for most RBMs. Approximately 30% speak to a medical professional (perhaps a technologist or billing specialist or nurse). Of the 30%, about half are resolved at this level. Of the remaining 15% of cases, there is an interaction with a physician with a decision to approve, reject, or cancel the study that is ordered (Michael Pentecost, personal communication, 2010).

The results from HealthHelp, published as part of an article on RBM impact by Levin and colleagues[25] (http://www.jacr.org/article/S1546-1440(09)00462-1/fulltext-article-footnote-1#article-footnote-1), are similar and can be found in **Table 2**.

Box 2
Major radiology benefits management companies (alphabetical)

AIM

Care to Care

CareCore National

HealthHelp

MedCurrent

MedSolutions

NIA

Table 2
Results from the radiology benefits management call center during 2008

	Requests (n)	Approved (%)	Request Withdrawn (%)	Examination Changed (%)	No Callback (%)	No Consensus (%)	Referred to Next Tier (%)
Tier 1	404,612	299,961 (74)	4164 (1)	—	—	—	100,487 (25)
Tier 2	100,487	82,598 (82)	4468 (4)	1736 (2)	1849 (2)	—	9836 (10)
Tier 3	9836	6406 (65)	1261 (13)	397 (4)	1620 (16)	152 (2)	—

Note: tier 1 is staffed by clinical service representatives, tier 2 by nurses, and tier 3 by subspecialized radiologists.
Data from HealthHelp, Inc. (Houston, TX).

From the data found in **Table 1**, there is an overall rate of study withdrawn or changed of 4%; 9833 requests were withdrawn in 2008. Given a Medicare global fee rate of (an inexpensive study) $280 for a noncontrast head CT, this would result in savings of $2,753,240.

NIA also monitors the quality of the imaging centers to which its managed patients are directed. The age of the scanners, whether they are American College of Radiology (ACR) certified, and the owner of the scanner are scrutinized. Self-referral is addressed by identifying those imaging centers that reside within clinical offices or are listed as being owned wholly or in part by the ordering physicians. NIA keeps records as to whether an ordering physicians have a specific financial interest in the imaging center to which they direct their patients.

Although many RBMs follow ACR guidelines for what studies are appropriate for which indications, some, like NIA, use proprietary software (Informa) to derive their own set of guidelines that may supplement the ACR guidelines or may be based on evidence-based literature that may contradict ACR guidelines. These guidelines are reviewed periodically by the Imaging Advisory Committee and the physician leadership of NIA. Public display of these guidelines based on individual insurance programs provides transparency in NIA's processes. From NIA's RadMD Web site (www. radmd.com), an insurer, an imaging modality, and a specific imaging study can be chosen.

In the case of disputes between referring physicians and the initial call center contact/nurse/physician/radiologist expert chain of command in an RBM, some RBMs use a third-party arbiter such as MCMC (Managing Care. Managing Claims. Quincy, MA). MCMC provides independent evidence-based peer reviews from a panel of paid medical consultants with rapid turnaround times. The likelihood of coming to such an independent arbitration is low in the processes of most RBMs. Personal intervention by radiologist medical directors usually solves any disagreements on imaging test appropriateness.

What are the controversial techniques that RBMs may use that lead some to question their intermediary function? Some physicians aggressively disdain the attitudes of RBMs about self-referral. Cardiologists and orthopedic surgeons in particular think that the patient convenience and guarantee of compliance when studies are performed directly in a physician's office (1-stop shop) warrant approval of these studies. Many RBMs use a strategy also used by some insurers in that they only approve studies at sites where at least 5 modalities of imaging (eg, MR imaging, CT, ultrasound, mammography, nuclear medicine) are offered.[26,27] This strategy has an effect of preventing self-referral sites of physicians that only have higher RVUs (CT and MR imaging) but may also exclude some smaller outpatient radiology groups that do not have the means to provide all modalities because of lack of resources for purchasing the machinery or lack of expertise for reading all studies. RBMs may also engage in the privileging of radiology providers to perform and interpret imaging studies.[27] Site inspections to ensure that equipment, software, and safety standards are maintained may also be performed by RBMs.

RBMs may also keep profiles of referring physicians and practice patterns to identify those physicians who are heavier or indiscriminate users of high-RVU procedures.[27] These physician offices may go through algorithms for approval that have more resistance points that physicians who have better records of ordering less frequent and/or more appropriate (by RBM standards) studies. The RBMs realize that the hassle factor of approval of studies may be effective in having physicians defer some studies and/or change practice patterns. Hence the RBMs may place obstacles before physicians who have a track record of abuse. RBMs are also paid incentives for reducing use. In some cases, bonuses may be linked to individual performance with the organization for ratios of denied or approved studies. Preferential treatment to those physicians who are low-use orderers may include higher fees and bonuses paid to those physicians.[27] In some cases, the pressure of performance (being monitored by the RBM) and the overall hassle factor may lead to reductions in ordering imaging studies.[28]

The impact of RBMs on use is couched in some secrecy because of the conflict sometimes perceived between referring physicians and RBMs and patients and RBMs. However, a July 2008 white paper by AHIP of Washington, DC (http://www.ahip.org/content/default.aspx?docid=24057), estimated that the use of RBMs reduced imaging expenditures by 10% to 20%.[27,29] Based on these data, the Medicare Payment Advisory Commission (MedPAC) has recommended that RBMs be examined for use in the Medicare system.

The AHIP white paper (p.7) states that:

...After implementation of a radiology benefit management program, health insurance plans report use rates have dropped the annual trend significantly, ranging from 20% to greater than 100%...

The reference for this claim is not the peer reviewed literature, but is listed in the white paper as:

Interviews conducted with health insurance plans for US Government Accountability Office.

Later in the same white paper (p. 8), the AHIP states that "radiology benefit management programs are able to achieve 10 to 20 percent reduction in actual expenditures; while mature programs can hold annual costs trends between 5 and 7 percent."[28]

The AHIP goes on to state that:

Several health insurance plans have reported reductions in the average growth of use from 25% to 1% after a radiology benefit management program was implemented. Others report an 82% decrease in use of inappropriate imaging and reductions of up to $2.00 per member per month over two years.

The reference for this statement is also difficult to critically assess because it is cited as "Interviews with health plans as reported in US Government Accountability Office. Medicare Part B imaging services: rapid spending growth and shift to physician offices indicate need for CMS to consider additional management practices. GAO-08-452. Washington, DC. June 2008."[30]

Nonetheless, these numbers are offered frequently by insurers for RBM impact.

The Government Accountability Office report also recounts the following scenario with respect to impact of RBMs:

An official at one plan told us about the plan's experience using RBM-performed prior authorization. To control rapid spending growth, the plan contracted with an RBM in the late 1990s to perform prior authorization for advanced imaging services. After 3 years, when expenditures for these services stopped growing, the plan discontinued using the RBM for prior authorization, assuming that a lasting change had been achieved in physicians' ordering of the services. However, over the subsequent 3 years, annual growth in imaging services climbed to more than 10 percent, on average. In 2006, the plan reinstated the RBM's prior authorization program and 6 months after implementation, growth had again declined to single digits.[30]

One point to make about RBMs is the subjective nature of the review process. The neuroradiology team at Thomas Jefferson University hospital works in collaboration with HealthHelp LLC in a utilization management program.[31] Friedman and Smith[32] reported a 2-fold variability between neuroradiology use reviewers in withdrawal rates when consulting with the referring physician about a potentially nonindicated study. The withdrawal rates (which include canceled or changed studies) varied from 12.8% to 23.5% between 5 neuroradiologists. More specifically, canceled studies ranged from 7.6% to 18.0% between the 5. When subspecialty fellows' rates were surveyed, a 4-fold rate of withdrawal of the ordered study was observed, ranging from 6.8% to 27.2%, and canceled studies varied by a factor of 7. Even though the rules under which decisions were supposed to be made were identical across these utilization management (UM) radiologists, there was wide variation in rejections. This finding points out the subjectivity of the gatekeeper function that could be at play by professional reviewers in RBMs. Friedman and Smith[32] state that "...the personality characteristics of each neuroradiologist (reviewer) are more likely to come into play in this situation: for example, qualities such as persuasiveness, persistence, and tolerance for potential conflict become important..."[32] These traits are exaggerated when fellows, not attendings, are in the sentinel role, as noted earlier. The investigators conclude that "...it is essential that radiologists with the most appropriate skill sets play key roles in the delivery of UM services."[32] This opinion is subjective.

Whether the promised savings of RBMs exceed the administrative expense of the RBM interaction has not been fully explored to date. There is a cost that the RBMs charge, but those rates are not transparent. The net impact that RBMs have on the total health system was recently explored by Lee and colleagues.[33] The costs of the RBMs are listed in **Box 3**.

Savings are borne by (1) decreasing use, (2) reduced out-of-pocket expenses with fewer procedures, and (3) avoidance of downstream costs from equivocal findings on imaging studies.

When Lee and colleagues[33] assumed an RBM denial rate of 12.5%, a physician-staff interaction time for preauthorization of 20 minutes with the RBM, 20 minutes for an initial and final appeal, an hourly rate of $15 for staff time and $117/h of physician time, and insurance payments of $380 per imaging study managed by the RBM, for a 100,000-member private insurance plan, the cost savings were $640,263. To be revenue neutral, the per member per month (PMPM) RBM charge would be $0.38. Denial rates of 5%, 10%, and 15% would result in a zero-sum gain if RBM charges were $0.20, $0.40, and $0.60 PMPM, respectively. The point is that the RBM-related costs are shifted to physicians and their staff and result in less of a cost reduction to the whole society than was initially expected.[33] RBMs may save money for a payer but increase the cost of providing health care to patients at the system level. As a whole, the preauthorization process is estimated to have costs of $31 billion for nurses, physicians, and office staff.[34]

Most recently, NIA commissioned Milliman, Inc to estimate the savings that could be achieved if RBMs controlled all Medicare fee-for-service products (which currently covers 34.7 million patients) over the 10-year period from 2011 to 2020, assuming the reductions that have been achieved through the use of NIA and 1 of its competitors.[24] The Milliman report calculated savings of $13 billion to $24 billion over a 10-year period, shared between CMS and the Medicare beneficiary. Milliman assumed a 3% increase in usage each year in its calculations, which were restricted to CT, MR imaging, and PET. Their second assumption, based on historical data, was that, on average, 89.8% of CT, 82.6% of MR, and 80.2% of PET requests were approved for performance by the RBM. A similar analysis developed and validated by Dobson Davanzo & Associates, LLC, and commissioned by MedSolutions in 2009 projected savings of up to $18 billion over 10 years (http://www.medsolutions.com/news/7-16-09.html).

An ACR white paper on RBM best practices can be found at: http://www.acr.org/Hidden/Economics/FeaturedCategories/WhatsNew/Attachments/ACR-RBMA-RBM-Guidelines.aspx.

COMPUTERIZED OEDS

Computerized decision support ideally would be universally applied across all ordering environments. It would provide immediate feedback to requesting physicians about the appropriateness of the given order based on patient clinical history and findings matched to a well-respected authority (in this case the ACR Appropriateness Criteria). It would take no more time for the ordering office staff/physician to request than simply calling in the order. OEDS would provide reports of physician ordering patterns and would provide references for substantiating its recommendations, allowing physician education. It would increase 24 × 7 × 365. It would be updated to current thought and evidence-based medicine research. Expense reduction would be achieved through the elimination of redundant or inappropriate orders, call centers, and expenses associated with commissioning RBMs.[35]

In the internal medicine literature, clinical decision support systems have led to marked reductions in medication order errors, improvement in medication prescribing behavior, and decreases in adverse drug events.[36] The cost savings for implementing such a system for prescribing medications outweighed the development and maintenance costs of the system, and patient safety is enhanced.

Early adopters of the concept of computerized decision support to direct clinicians to order the appropriate study for a specific indication include Nuance (Burlington, MA) HealthCare's RadPort (**Box 4**). The guidelines for Nuance's product are based on the ACR Appropriateness Criteria and

---

Box 3
Costs of RBMs

1. Payers paying the RBM for services

2. Physicians for time and staff to comply with RBM procedures

3. Patients who must self-pay for services denied by RBMs

4. Any delays in diagnosis or treatment incurred by RBM process

5. Loss of efficiency by clinicians to make diagnosis without imaging

are vetted through a committee in association with Massachusetts General Hospital. RadPort satisfies precertification requirements when accepted by a network of health care payers. RadPort software is installed at 12 sites as of late 2011. The back-end analytics component of the software is called RadCube.

The other main player in decision support software, Medicalis, also has links to the Harvard Medical System. Medicalis was founded in 1999 as a joint venture with Brigham and Women's Hospital, to design and implement a Web-native solution for the delivery of clinical decision support to ordering physicians. It is currently based in San Francisco, California, as an independent corporation and separated from the Brigham and Women's Hospital in 2002.

Medicalis has a current client base that includes Partners HealthCare, Medica, Geisinger Health System, Marshfield Clinic, Weill Cornell Medical College/New York Presbyterian, and the University of Pennsylvania Hospital. It recently deployed DSCloud, a product that is offered nationwide for clinical decision support and has been selected for a CMS Medicare Imaging Demonstration (MID) project.

MedCurrent's OrderRight software is another player in the market. The company has headquarters in Los Angeles, California, and Toronto, Ontario. Although the company has been around since 2002, it debuted its decision support software in 2010. The Institute for Clinical Systems Improvement (ICSI) in Bloomington, Minnesota, supports clinical decision support with a pilot project in Minnesota. Health insurance providers in Minnesota are now paying to implement clinical decision support statewide and to make it mandatory for ICSI members. The state used the ICSI software to improve the diagnostic usefulness of scans ordered, reduce patient exposure to radiation, increase provider efficiency, aid in provider-patient shared decision making, and save Minnesota $84 million over 3 years (http://www.health careitnews.com/news/nuance-icsi-aim-prevent-unnescessary-imaging-tests). ICSI's pilot project on decision support showed that, although dealing with RBMs to respond to prior-authorization restrictions took an extra 10 minutes of time per study ordered, with computerized decision support it only took an extra 10 seconds.

Since then, many institutions have experimented with creating their own algorithm and homegrown decision support order entry systems. Thus the market has not really consolidated around any 1 product in the decision support market.

What are the basic commonalities of the OEDS systems? Most require physician order input either by clinical symptoms or by ICD-9 code. Most rely on appropriateness criteria guidelines like those vetted by the ACR. Most provide a flowchart that directs the clinician toward a particular modality and a decision about whether to request contrast media. In most cases, ordering physicians are not faced with a hard-stop command but have the possibility to override the judgment of the computer algorithm to order the study they wish. Some do have a point at which human interaction is required to override the recommendations of the decision support algorithm, which is a disincentive. If clinicians abide by the algorithm, they get to order their study without hesitation and they are finished. If they do not acquiesce, they have to spend time on the phone and justify their resistance to the recommended study and do not get immediate gratification.

CMS entered the OEDS debate with a call for pilot project submissions. The Medicare Imaging Demonstration project study will consider ordering results for the 11 advanced imaging procedures most commonly paid for by Medicare: CT of the brain, sinus, thorax, abdomen, lumbar spine, and pelvis; MR imaging of the brain, lumbar spine, shoulder, and knee; and single-photon emission CT myocardial perfusion imaging (http://www.cms.gov/DemoProjectsEvalRpts/downloads/Medicare_Imaging_Demonstration.pdf). CMS selected the Brigham & Women's Hospital, Henry Ford Health System, Maine Medical Center-Physician Hospital Organization, University of Wisconsin-Madison, and NIA as the sites for the pilot projects to assess the impact that decision support systems have on the appropriateness and use of advanced medical imaging services ordered for beneficiaries in original fee-for-service Medicare.

An example from the article by Blackmore and colleagues[37] is a representative example of a decision tree for OEDS (**Fig. 3**).

The impact of adding a decision support intervention such as the one outlined in **Fig. 3** on several neuroradiology studies was shown in the graph (**Fig. 4**) by Blackmore and colleagues.[37] Note the immediate impact on usage after the computer-based learning tool was implemented.

When the Massachusetts General Hospital implemented its OEDS system, the order entry

---

MRI Back Exam

Exam Requested*	

☐ mr cspine   ☐ mr tspine   ☐ mr lspine

☐ mr cspine w/ w/o contrast   ☐ mr tspine w/ w/o contrast   ☐ mr lspine w/ w/o contrast

Current Weight*   [　　　　] ⦿ lbs ○ kg Max Table Weight 200 kg/441 lbs

ICD9 Code(s)   [　　　　　　]

Indications (select all that apply):*

☐ **Motor deficit (781.99)**
☐ **Unremitting pain despite 6 weeks of appropriate therapy**
   (appropriate therapy is defined as 2 weeks of NSAIDs AND advice to stay active AND documentation of lack of improvement)
   Document in relevant history field and apply appropriate ICD 9 code
☐ **Strong suspicion of systemic disease**
   Document in relevant history field and apply appropriate ICD 9 code
☐ **Neurogenic Claudication(435.9)**
☐ **Cauda Equina(344.60)**
☐ **Upper motor neuron findings:** use myelopathy codes
   ☐ **Unspecified Region (722.70)**
   ☐ **Cervical (722.71)**
   ☐ **Thoracic (722.72)**
   ☐ **Lumbar (722.73)**
☐ **Significant trauma or fall**
   Document in relevant history field and apply appropriate ICD 9 code
☐ **Consult has been performed by physical medicine.**

NOTE: A spine MRI will likely not be helpful for the patient with back or neck pain if none of these indications are present. The Spine Clinic physician on call will provide help by phone and offer a same day visit to assist in care of the patient. Text page (spine clinic page number) on V-Net and enter the following message: "Dr. --- wishes to speak with you about a patient with neck/back pain in whom an MRI is not indicated. Please call (pager number of ordering provider).

Additional Information (Rule Out, History, Symptoms)   [　　　　　　　　　　　　　　]

Is this patient uncomfortable in enclosed spaces?*
○ No
○ Yes, Uncomfortable, but can tolerate exam
○ Yes, Oral medication provided and ride home confirmed
○ Yes, Moderate Sedation Required

Able to lie on back for 30 min?*
○ Yes
○ No, can not lie on back. Oral medication provided and ride home confirmed
○ No, can not lie on back. Moderate sedation required.

Previous metal worker?*   ○ No ○ Yes

Fig. 3. A decision tree for OEDS. (*From* Blackmore CC, Mecklenburg RS, Kaplan GS. Effectiveness of clinical decision support in controlling inappropriate imaging. J Am Coll Radiol 2011;8:19–25; with permission.)

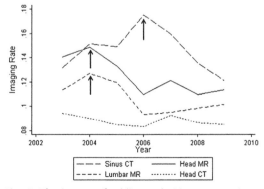

Fig. 4. The impact of adding a decision support intervention (*Arrow* marks the date of intervention). (*From* Blackmore CC, Mecklenburg RS, Kaplan GS. Effectiveness of clinical decision support in controlling inappropriate imaging. J Am Coll Radiol 2011;8:19–25; with permission.)

software provided an appropriateness score of 1 to 9 based on the ACR's Appropriateness Criteria and indication and procedure pairs developed by a consensus panel of Massachusetts General Hospital radiologists, primary care physicians, and specialist clinicians. The scoring system for evaluating the appropriateness of studies ordered by its referring physician directs the clinicians from low-usefulness (inappropriate) studies toward higher (most appropriate) usefulness studies. The results of implementing this system were impressive. The percentage of low-usefulness examinations declined from 6% to 2%. The highest number of low-usefulness examinations were CT scans and MR imaging of the spine overall. Primary care physicians accounted for some of the steepest declines in inappropriate low-usefulness

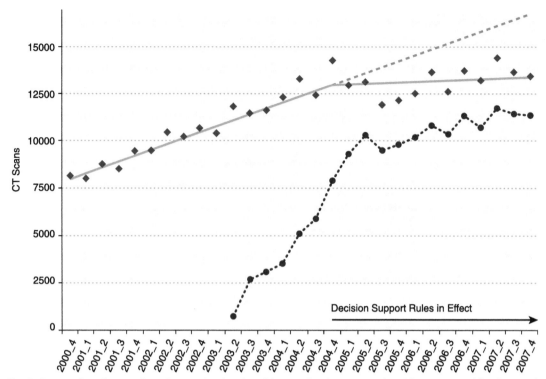

Fig. 5. Scatterplot of outpatient CT examination (y-axis) per calendar quarter (x-axis) represented by diamonds. The solid line represents the linear component of the piecewise regression with break point at quarter 4 of 2004 and accounting for outpatient visit numbers. The dashed line shows projected linear growth without implementation of a radiology order entry and decision support system. Dotted line and circles depict the number of CT examinations ordered through computer order entry. Appropriateness feedback was started in quarter 4 of 2004 and continued throughout the study (*arrow* at *lower right*).

studies, especially if they, and not their office staff, interacted with the OEDS. Office staff may simply and blindly follow orders to request the study their boss has demanded and override the system.[38]

In a follow-up study by Sistrom and colleagues[39] of ordering patterns from October to December 2007, the research team noted a substantial decrease in the growth rate of high-RVU CT, MR

Table 3
Necessary criteria for an effective electronic decision support recommendation tool

Evidence Based	Standards Collated from National Societies Meeting Appropriateness Criteria
Consensus driven	Radiologist, institutional, and nonradiologist input
Effective	Improves clinical and financial outcomes
Transparent	Standard recommendation methodology open to stakeholders
Adaptable	Meets specific needs of organizations and clinical practice
Iterative	Can be updated as new best practices become available
Reproducible	Can be implemented across diverse organizations
Standardized	Multiorganizational conformity to accepted best practices; recommendation language standardized with macros
Easy to use	Seamless integration into existing information system platforms; fast, and data input minimized to critical information
Data mining	Analysis of quantity, cost, benchmarking to institutional and national data
Educational	Opportunity to educate stakeholders to current and future best practices

Reproduced from Boland GW, Thrall JH, Gazelle GS, et al. Decision support for radiologist report recommendations. J Am Coll Radiol 2011;8(12):819–23; with permission.

imaging, and ultrasound imaging studies (MR, CT, and ultrasound). Although outpatient visits increased at a compound annual growth rate of nearly 5%, the corresponding CT, MR, and ultrasound growth rates decreased from 12%, 12%, and 9% before implementing OEDS to 1%, 7%, and 4%, respectively, after OEDS use (Fig. 5). It is hoped that the impact is more what Sistrom and colleagues[39] call an educational factor as the clinician learns the appropriate test for a set of clinical symptoms, rather than just a gatekeeper factor putting obstacles in the way of the ordering physicians. The educational factor is more long lasting.

The benefits of OEDS were also shown in work by Solberg and colleagues[40] in reducing use. Charts were audited for MR imaging and CT scans of the head, and MR imaging of the lumbar spine before and after implementation of an OEDS system. Decision support was associated with a 20% to 36% decrease in spine MR imaging and head CT orders, but no change in the number head MR imaging orders.[40] On chart review, the rate of positive studies was unchanged after implementing the OEDS program. Thus the investigators concluded that there was no substantive change in quality of patient care despite the

Table 4
Summary of advantages and disadvantages of RBMs versus OEDS

	RBM	OEDS
Advantages	1. Knowledgeable and focused 2. Prevent abuse 3. Prevent duplication, redundancy 4. Advise physicians 5. Generally radiology-specific employees 6. Better than MCO nonradiology operatives 7. Keep patients out of self-referral and nonaccredited facilities 8. Allow for third-party adjudication 9. Promote access to affordable, quality services	1. Effective to help control inappropriate use 2. Transparent to clinicians by supported criteria 3. Yields reproducible answers 4. Efficient; no added costs or time, does not disrupt workflow 5. Enhances patient safety, decreasing risks of allergy, radiation 6. Flexible, providing choice when appropriate, for extenuating circumstances 7. Educational to improve ordering patterns for future 8. Developmental: evolves with new technologies 9. 24 × 7 × 365
Disadvantages	1. Adding an intermediary adds costs 2. Interferes with doctor-patient relationship 3. Adds hurdles/time to request studies 4. Motivation is to save money not expedite patient care 5. May be owned by radiologists with vested interests to direct flow-constrain competition 6. Often does not have access to prior other-network studies 7. Cannot deliver prior studies to radiologists from outside the system 8. Often lack of access to inpatient studies, ED studies, low RVU examinations 9. Push to lowest-cost imaging centers not best quality 10. Focus only on expensive tests 11. Not always available 24 × 7 for preauthorization	1. No teeth 2. No hard stop 3. Impersonal 4. Not knowledgeable or flexible enough 5. No physician interaction 6. Radiologist based and produced, therefore potentially biased 7. Not incentivized to control cost 8. Arbitrary without individualization possible

Abbreviation: MCO, Managed Care Organization.

reduction in high-RVU studies performed based on using OEDS appropriateness criteria.

Boland and colleagues[41] recently suggested that decision support should be applied to radiologists when they make recommendations for further imaging. In cases in which an initial study is non-diagnostic or a lesion needs to be followed, Boland and colleagues[41] recommend that appropriateness guidelines be applied to the radiologist's recommendations for the next study. Rather than leaving it to the radiologists' preferences for how they would like to pursue a lesion, these investigators argue that the report and recommendation should be driven by national (ACR) or institutionally derived criteria via decision support software integrated into speech recognition software dictation systems. When recommendations for further imaging for an incidental finding, for example, are contemplated, the radiologist would navigate through a series of decision trees so that the right next test is suggested. In this way, claims of radiology self-referral could be addressed. This method would be point-of-care best-practice radiology reporting decision support.

In the same article, Boland and colleagues[41] described the factors that would make a good OEDS system, which are summarized in Table 3.

SUMMARY

The health care community is struggling with how to regulate itself with regard to the increases in imaging use that often accompany new and advanced technologies. The tendency to overorder stems in part from patient demand, medicolegal considerations, a desire to eliminate the potential for mistakes highlighted in the Institute of Medicine report, and, in some cases, motivation for financial gain by self-referrers. The radiology community thinks that it can provide the solutions that will eliminate unnecessary and inappropriate imaging studies, and several institutions have therefore embraced computerized decision support tied to electronic physician order entry (POE). This alternative to having external oversight by RBMs has reduced the overheads associated with it and eliminates the intermediary function of the RBM approval process. However, its effectiveness has yet to be proved across different practice patterns outside academic centers, and its cost for smaller imaging groups without sophisticated IT support and electronic POE may be prohibitive. RBMs have largely been embraced by payers because of their record of reducing high-RVU numbers and their ability to prevent abuse of the system, as could occur with an OEDS system that does not have direct human monitoring. By virtue of human one-on-one interaction, RBMs can be more flexible than OEDS systems and the interaction is more likely to influence practice patterns. Until head-to-head competition between RBMs and OEDS leads to a definitive winner, both solutions will likely grow in the United States health care system (Table 4).

REFERENCES

1. Mitchell JM. Utilization trends for advanced imaging procedures: evidence from individuals with private insurance coverage in California. Med Care 2008;46:460–6.
2. Bhargavan M, Sunshine JH. Utilization of radiology services in the United States: levels and trends in modalities, regions, and populations. Radiology 2005;234:824–32.
3. Hillman BJ, Joseph CA, Mabry MR, et al. Frequency and costs of diagnostic imaging in office practice—a comparison of self-referring and radiologist-referring physicians. N Engl J Med 1990;323:1604–8.
4. Radecki SE, Steele JP. Effect of on-site facilities on use of diagnostic radiology by non-radiologists. Invest Radiol 1990;25:190–3.
5. Hillman BJ, Olson GT, Griffith PE, et al. Physicians' utilization and charges for outpatient diagnostic imaging in a Medicare population. JAMA 1992;268:2050–4.
6. Kouri BE, Parsons RG, Alpert HR. Physician self-referral for diagnostic imaging: review of the empiric literature. AJR Am J Roentgenol 2002;179:843–50.
7. Maitino AJ, Levin DC, Parker L, et al. Practice patterns of radiologists and nonradiologists in utilization of noninvasive diagnostic imaging among the Medicare population 1993-1999. Radiology 2003;228(3):795–801.
8. Litt AW, Ryan DR, Batista D, et al. Relative procedure intensity with self-referral and radiologist referral: extremity radiography. Radiology 2005;235:142–7.
9. Gazelle GS, Halpern EF, Ryan HS, et al. Utilization of diagnostic medical imaging: comparison of radiologist referral versus same-specialty referral. Radiology 2007;245:517–22.
10. Levin DC, Rao VM. Turf wars in radiology: updated evidence on the relationship between self-referral and the overutilization of imaging. J Am Coll Radiol 2008;5:806–10.
11. Levin DC, Rao VM, Parker L, et al. Recent shifts in place of service for noninvasive diagnostic imaging: have hospitals missed an opportunity? J Am Coll Radiol 2009;6:96–9.
12. Agarwal R, Levin DC, Parker L, et al. Trends in PET scanner ownership and leasing by nonradiologist physicians. J Am Coll Radiol 2010;7(3):187–91.

13. Levin DC, Rao VM, Parker L, et al. Medicare payments for noninvasive diagnostic imaging are now higher to nonradiologist physicians than to radiologists. J Am Coll Radiol 2011;8:26–32.

14. Dunnick NR, Applegate KE, Arenson RL. The inappropriate use of imaging studies: a report of the 2004 Intersociety Conference. J Am Coll Radiol 2005;2(5):401–6.

15. Levin DC, Intenzo CM, Rao VM, et al. Comparison of recent utilization trends in radionuclide myocardial perfusion imaging among radiologists and cardiologists. J Am Coll Radiol 2005;2(10):821–4.

16. Mitchell JM. The prevalence of physician self-referral arrangements after Stark II: evidence from advanced diagnostic imaging. Health Aff (Millwood) 2007;26:w415–24.

17. Levin DC, Rao VM, Parker L, et al. Recent trends in utilization rates of abdominal imaging: the relative roles of radiologists and nonradiologist physicians. J Am Coll Radiol 2008;5(6):744–7.

18. Babiarz LS, Yousem DM, Parker L, et al. Utilization rates of neuroradiology across neuroscience specialties in the private office setting: who owns or leases the scanners on which studies are performed? AJNR Am J Neuroradiol 2011;33(1):43–8.

19. Hendee WR, Becker GJ, Borgstede JP, et al. Addressing overutilization in medical imaging. Radiology 2010;257(1):240–5.

20. Oguz KK, Yousem DM, Deluca T, et al. Effect of emergency department CT on neuroimaging case volume and positive scan rates. Acad Radiol 2002;9(9):1018–24.

21. Lehnert BE, Bree RL. Analysis of appropriateness of outpatient CT and MRI referred from primary care clinics at an academic medical center: how critical is the need for improved decision support? J Am Coll Radiol 2010;7(3):192–7.

22. American Health Insurance Plans. Ensuring Quality Through Appropriate Use of Diagnostic Imaging. Washington, DC: America's HealthInsurance Plans; 2011.

23. Stein C. Code red partners program aims to rein in skyrocketing costs of diagnostic imaging. Boston Globe 2003.

24. Anne Jackson E. Potential savings for fee-for-service Medicare from radiology benefits management programs. Milliman. Available at: http://www.niahealthcare.com/media/430357/potential-savings-to-medicare-ffs-from-rbm-programs.pdf. Accessed July 13, 2011.

25. Levin DC, Bree RL, Rao VM, et al. A prior authorization program of a radiology benefits management company and how it has affected utilization of advanced diagnostic imaging. J Am Coll Radiol 2010;7:33–8.

26. Rothenberg BM, Korn A. The opportunities and challenges posed by the rapid growth of diagnostic imaging. J Am Coll Radiol 2005;2:407–10.

27. Mitchell JM, Lagalia RR. Controlling the escalating use of advanced imaging: the role of radiology benefit management programs. Med Care Res Rev 2009 Jun;66(3):339–51.

28. Reinke T. New imaging controls strict, but may be easier on doctors. Manag Care 2007. Available at: http://www.managedcaremag.com/archives/0711/0711.imaging.html. Accessed July 8, 2008.

29. Iglehart JK. Health insurers and medical-imaging policy — a work in progress. N Engl J Med 2009;360:1030–7.

30. Rapid spending growth and shift to physician offices indicate need for CMS to consider additional management practices. GAO-08-452. Washington, DC. 2008. Available at: http://www.gao.gov/new.items/d08452.pdf. Accessed January 3, 2012.

31. Friedman DP, Smith NS, Bree RL, et al. Experience of an academic neuroradiology division participating in a utilization management program. J Am Coll Radiol 2009;6:119–24.

32. Friedman DP, Smith NS. Variability in study withdrawal rates among academic neuroradiologists participating in a radiology utilization management program. J Am Coll Radiol 2011;8:716–9.

33. Lee DW, Rawson JV, Wade SW. Radiology benefit managers: cost saving or cost shifting? J Am Coll Radiol 2011;8:393–401.

34. Casalino LP, Nicholson S, Gans DN, et al. What does it cost physician practices to interact with health insurance plans? Health Aff (Millwood) 2009;28(4):w533–43.

35. Hardy K. Decision support for Rad reports. Radiology Today 2010;11:16.

36. Kaushal R, Shojania KG, Bates DW. Effects of computerized physician order entry and clinical decision support systems on medication safety: a systematic review. Arch Intern Med 2003;163:1409–16.

37. Blackmore CC, Mecklenburg RS, Kaplan GS. Effectiveness of clinical decision support in controlling inappropriate imaging. J Am Coll Radiol 2011;8:19–25.

38. Rosenthal DI, Weilburg JB, Schultz T, et al. Radiology order entry with decision support: initial clinical experience. J Am Coll Radiol 2006;3:799–806.

39. Sistrom CL, Dang PA, Weilburg JB, et al. Effect of computerized order entry with integrated decision support on the growth of outpatient procedure volumes: seven-year time series analysis. Radiology 2009;251(1):147–55.

40. Solberg LI, Wei F, Butler JC, et al. Effects of electronic decision support on high-tech diagnostic imaging orders and patients. Am J Manag Care 2010;16(2):102–6.

41. Boland GW, Thrall JH, Gazelle GS, et al. Decision support for radiologist report recommendations. J Am Coll Radiol 2011;8(12):819–23.

Teleradiology

William G. Bradley Jr, MD, PhD

KEYWORDS

• Teleradiology • Radiology • Imaging • Subspecialists

KEY POINTS

- Picture archiving and communication systems and the Internet are the key enablers of teleradiology.
- More than half of the radiology groups in the United States are covered by a nighthawk service.
- Teleradiology is improving patient care by bringing subspecialist interpretations to small and rural practices.

The times they are a-changin'
—(Robert A. Zimmerman aka Bob Dylan, 1964)

Teleradiology has probably been around in one form or another since there were radiologists. In the early days of the last century, plain films taken in physicians' offices were sometimes couriered to radiologists for expert interpretation. In the early days of magnetic resonance (MR) imaging almost 3 decades ago, I received images by FedEx and interpreted them remotely before dictating a report or calling the referring radiologist. Although these methods of dissociating the site of image acquisition from the site of interpretation could be called teleradiology, a more modern definition would involve sending digital images over the Internet. With the widespread implementation of picture archiving and communication systems (PACS) and increasing Internet bandwidth, teleradiology for nighttime coverage and daytime subspecialty reads became possible approximately 20 years ago. This article reviews the history of teleradiology with parallels to the changing times of radiology as a specialty and the recent advent of the Digital Age. It examines the bright and dark sides of teleradiology with regard to lifestyle, quality interpretations, and potential for commoditization and predatory practices.

A little more than 50 years ago, radiologists were viewed as ancillary.[1] They did not provide nighttime or weekend coverage; they just read out whatever accumulated during the off hours during the next business day. There was not much demand for them to provide after-hours readings because most clinical specialists thought they could read radiographs as well as radiologists. Most radiology groups consisted of fewer than 5 so-called utility infielders, interchangeable and generalists, who covered all the bases. Because it did not really matter who read what, they might have been considered to be a commodity. With the introduction of computed tomography (CT) and then MR imaging, most clinicians realized that they did need radiologists for the interpretation, and that they needed them 24/7. Add to this the trend toward increasing subspecialization, and the fellowship-trained radiologists were becoming part of the clinical team, and clearly not a commodity. Radiology groups were also tending to increase in size to adequately load the radiology subspecialists with work.

Radiology took a step backward with regard to commoditization with PACS.[2] Before full PACS implementation several years ago, our clinicians used to come down to the Radiology Department to discuss their cases. It was good for us because

Disclosures: William G. Bradley Jr is Professor and Chair of Radiology at UCSD. He is a former Board member, consultant, and stockholder of NightHawk Radiology Services, Coeur d'Alene, ID.
Department of Radiology, UCSD Medical Center, 402 Dickinson Street, Suite 454, San Diego, CA 92103-8224, USA
E-mail address: wgbradley@mail.ucsd.edu

Neuroimag Clin N Am 22 (2012) 511–517
doi:10.1016/j.nic.2012.05.001
1052-5149/12 $ – see front matter © 2012 Elsevier Inc. All rights reserved.

the clinicians either provided additional history, which might lead to a better diagnosis, or confirmed a diagnosis already made, which is important feedback about our image interpretation skills. In the process, we got to know each other. Over time, if we generally provided accurate interpretations, the clinician would make allowances if we subsequently made an error. Some clinicians wanted specific, personalized radiologists to review their cases. As mutual respect was developed, we found ourselves supporting each other on potentially contentious medical staff issues.

Now that PACS has been fully implemented, we rarely see our clinicians. They can see the images and read our reports in their offices, or in the clinics or on the floors of the medical center. What a time saving in a medical world where efficiency is paramount! The only time the referring physicians now call is when they disagree with a reading. They rarely come to the Radiology Department anymore because we can each access the same image on PACS from different locations to discuss over the phone. As a result, many of the clinicians cannot put a name to the face of many of our junior faculty, fellows, and residents (and vice versa). The camaraderie of the old days is gone and we are being increasingly commoditized. Furthermore, with increasing priority being placed on productivity, many radiologists do not even want to see or talk to the clinicians because it just slows them down with non-relative value unit (RVU)-producing work.[3] So although I do not disagree that teleradiology may contribute to commoditization, I think the real culprits are PACS and a culture that is becoming increasingly RVU-driven because of the decreasing reimbursement for radiology examinations and the desire to maintain income. When the only activity that provides bonuses is image interpretation productivity, and not friendly consults or attendance at tumor boards, radiologists adapt, and not necessarily in a good way.

This article discusses nighttime coverage and daytime subspecialty readings separately because they evolved independently.[2]

NIGHTTIME COVERAGE

Nighttime coverage has gone through 5 stages: (1) wake up and drive to the hospital, (2) wake up and read from home, (3) stay up at night and cover the emergency department (ED) internally, (4) outsource nighttime coverage to another US-based group working at night, and (5) outsource nighttime US coverage to another group working from offshore where it is daytime. Each of these stages is discussed from my personal experience.

Stage 1: Wake up and Drive into the Hospital

When I started practicing radiology in 1981, I had to drive my Toyota Celica into the hospital to read an emergency film. Each call resulted in about 2 hours of lost sleep, but at least we were awake by the time we arrived at the hospital. If the emergency room (ER) physician was reasonable, he would not call us in, except for extreme emergencies, such as a lateral cervical spine film for a broken neck (which turned out not to be as accurate as we thought once we started doing CT). The ER physicians would interpret the films at night, render treatment based on that interpretation and we would do the official reading the next morning. If there were a discrepancy, we would contact the ER and they would contact the patient if a different treatment was needed. This process was not exactly optimal patient care nor was it optimal for radiologists because they also had to work the next day after occasionally coming into the hospital the night before.

Stage 2: Wake up and Read from Home

In the mid-1980s, the first camera-on-a-stick teleradiology systems became available. I can remember our radiology group discussing whether we really wanted to adopt this technology because it might increase the number of times we were called at night. Although ER physicians might have a high threshold for calling us physically into the hospital, they would likely have a lower threshold to ask us to look at cases from a video unit in our homes. It turned out not to seriously affect the number of cases we were asked to see at night and it had the advantage (for us) that we could view the images at our bedside and not fully wake up. Reading a study while half asleep might not be thought to be optimal patient care, but this was the standard of care for the next decade, and I still dreaded my nights on call. It was the worst part of being a radiologist.

Stage 3: Stay up at Night and Cover ED Internally

In 1993, the Office of the Inspector General realized that management of patients at night was being based on the ER physician's interpretation of the images, not our interpretation the next morning. They decided that they would only pay for contemporaneous readings.[4] At that time, I was part of a 60-person radiology group (Memrad Medical Group, Inc.) that covered 7 hospitals in southern California. Memrad's president (Paul Berger, MD) realized that this ruling could potentially result in a significant loss of income to the group. If the ER physicians could read during the night, they would argue that they should be able to read during the day, which would decrease our income by 30%. Dr Berger was determined to provide contemporaneous readings, but to do it by having only 1 person stay up all night covering all 7 hospitals. This strategy was accomplished with expensive T1 lines and rudimentary teleradiology systems all feeding into 1 radiologist at the main hospital, Long Beach Memorial. Similar multihospital coverage was performed by other large private groups at about the same time.[5-8]

Our system went live on January 1, 1994. The night call was initially rotated among everybody in the group. My entry in the log book on January 4, 1994 was "worse night of my life since internship." In addition to getting several calls at once from different hospitals (where I did not work during the day), I was talking to ER physicians whom I did not know and who did not know me (commoditization). This system reduced the total number of nights we were on call and had the advantage that we were wide awake and probably rendering better contemporaneous readings than we had been doing half asleep at night from a video system at home. Because everyone in the group initially had to rotate through the system, we had neuroradiologists reading emergency body CT scans and body radiologists reading emergency brain MR images. We might have been awake but, because we were all subspecialized, we were not necessarily all skilled at reading emergency studies involving multiple organ systems.

It did not take long for the senior partners to start paying the junior partners (who were closer to residency and still utility infielders) to take their call. For those of us who were subspecialized, we argued that this was better patient care; the junior partners were also willing to work for the extra money. Market forces prevailed: after a few months the group paid the junior partners $1000 per night and gave them the next day off. Call generally occurred for a week at a time to minimize adjustments to the circadian rhythm. However, after about a year, even the junior partners burned out working 5 to 7 nights in a row, so we hired 4 radiologists whose job was to cover nights 1 week a month and cover days as internal locums 1 other week each month. They could take the other 2 weeks a month as vacation or they could work for more pay. The nighttime radiologists were dubbed "nighthawks." By extension, the same people working during the day became known as "dayhawks." However, there was still a premium for working at night; when I left Memrad for the University of California, San Diego (UCSD) in 2002, the nighthawks were each making 30% more than a full partner and were working 30% fewer hours.

Stage 4: Outsource Nighttime Coverage to Another US-Based Group Working at Night

When the 4 nighthawks were first hired, they dictated all the cases they saw at night. The argument was that there would be fewer films to read the next morning so we could cut the number of radiologists at a given hospital from, for example, 5 to 4, thereby covering the added cost of the nighthawks. This never happened. Those who had been used to 12 MR scans per day being a good day's work were reluctant to read more. Thus, to help pay for the nighthawks, we began covering for other groups, in effect insourcing their night calls. By relaxing the requirement that all studies be dictated by the nighthawk, we were able to cover more outside groups with just wet readings and bring in more outside income to cover the added cost of the nighthawks. At the same time, several commercial entities arose that only provided nighttime coverage to outside groups. These companies started providing coverage in the same state, then in the same region, and eventually throughout the United States. Radiologists found that they could make the same income just performing preliminary reports at night from home as going into a hospital where they had to deal with final detailed reports, referring clinicians, and even occasionally with patients. The process of commoditization was advancing further.

Stage 5: Outsource Nighttime US Coverage to Another Group Working from Offshore (Where it is Daytime)

In September 2000, we installed PACS in the MR imaging center at Long Beach Memorial. The next month I was lecturing in Xian, China, and was asked to read a neuro-MR imaging case from Long Beach by logging into our PACS unit over the Internet. When I called the neurosurgeon back home, it was the middle of the night there and the middle of the afternoon in China. I realized that radiologists no longer needed to be up at night. As a result of PACS and the Internet, they could read from anywhere in the world where it was daytime while it was nighttime in the United States. I discussed this with Paul Berger (who had retired from Memrad in 1995) and he turned the idea into NightHawk Radiology Services (NRS). Their first reading center was in Sydney, Australia, where the NightHawks read from midafternoon to midnight; a second center was subsequently established in Zurich, Switzerland where they read from 6 AM to midafternoon. By decoupling the nighttime US coverage from working at night, the extra pay premium for being up at night was obviated and compensation could be based on productivity and accuracy.[9]

One of the advantages of reading the most difficult emergency radiology studies from around the country is that the readers quickly become skilled at emergency radiology. Because most cases are dictated by the local group when previous studies and additional history are available the next morning, this led to a built-in quality assurance program. Any discrepancies between the wet reading and the final report were noted, providing feedback to both the nighthawk and the local radiologist. In addition to becoming skilled in ER radiology, the nighthawks were wide awake because it was their daytime. Reading from virtual centers of 20 radiologists or so scattered physically across the globe but linked electronically in an e-office, interesting cases could be shown around and second opinions sought on the more difficult cases.

In the last several years with the expansion of emergency CT scans, there has been an increasing demand for final reads in the middle of the night. Because the Centers for Medicare and Medicaid Services (CMS) requires that all Medicare and Medicaid studies be read from the United States (vs offshore),[10] the number of offshore teleradiologists has recently decreased relative to the number staying up at night in the United States. However, should CMS come to the realization that it does not matter where an American board–certified, state-licensed, hospital-credentialed radiologist is physically located, I expect the number of offshore American radiologists to again increase.

The original model for nighttime teleradiology was to provide preliminary wet reads that only involved sending the current CT. With a limited amount of data being transmitted, a stat report could be expected back within 20 to 30 minutes. With the trend to final reads, it has been pointed out that teleradiologists are at a disadvantage because they do not have access to the same resources that on-site radiologists have, namely prior imaging examinations, radiology information system (for prior reports) and hospital information system (for laboratory reports). Although this may be a problem today, the likely increase in bandwidth in the next several years should largely obviate it as a disadvantage.

It is important to stress that these are American trained and licensed physicians reading from offshore. There are plenty of excellent offshore radiologists who were not trained in the United States and do not have their American Boards who would love to read for us. Because radiology training is currently not standardized in other parts of the world and they have not taken our American Board of Radiology certification examination, it is difficult to know how competent they are. This is 1 of the reasons that American payers only pay for American trained and boarded radiologists. Such offshore American trained radiologists occasionally put their names on hundreds of reports per hour that were interpreted by radiologists who do not have their American Boards. This practice is called "ghost reading" and constitutes Medicare fraud.

Several years ago, our Dean insisted that the UCSD Radiology Department provide 24/7 attending readings to rule out pulmonary embolism and appendicitis. Realizing that they might be up half the night when they were on call, the chest and body faculty members threatened to resign en masse. The 30 or so Fellows at UCSD (all Board-certified utility infielders) eventually agreed to cover from 5 PM to 11 PM and we contracted with NightHawk (now vRad) to cover from 11 PM to 7 AM. The NRS radiologists who covered us all had California medical licenses and were credentialed on our medical staff as attendings.

Although there were 120 radiologists working as independent contractors for NightHawk during this time, only a small subset of them routinely covered UCSD, So our residents are covered by almost the same group of NightHawks from night to night.[11] Thus, the residents and ER doctors became familiar with the names on the reports or the voice on the other end of the phone. Although, superficially, this might look like commoditization, it is no more of a commodity than we currently have with PACS and (in academics) with residents and fellows coming and going.

At the time of this writing, more than half the hospitals in the United States use a nighttime service for coverage.[12] Although this may be driven by the desire for an easy lifestyle by radiologists, it could be argued that readings are more accurate when provided by fully awake emergency radiology subspecialists. As a result, off-site teleradiology continues to increase and is spreading to daytime subspecialty readings.

TELERADIOLOGY FOR DAYTIME SUBSPECIALTY READINGS

The growth of CT and MR imaging in the past 30 years has led to an increasing need for subspecialization. When I did my (3-year) residency in the late 1970s at the University of California, San Francisco (UCSF), there was a greater emphasis on barium studies than on CT. The Body Imaging fellowship during that period at UCSF was 50% fluoro and 50% CT. As CT and, subsequently, MR imaging became more advanced, it became virtually impossible for a general radiologist to be proficient at all cross-sectional imaging, let alone all radiology. Because CT has now essentially replaced the physical examination in the ED, subspecialty readings are required quickly and accurately on a 24/7 basis.

In an ideal situation, all subspecialty clinicians would be served by fellowship-trained subspecialty radiologists with whom they interact face to face on a daily basis. If this is not possible, a compromise is necessary. Either the local subspecialty clinicians need to interact with local general radiologists or they need to interact with subspecialist radiologists at a distance by teleradiology. I argue that the latter is preferable for patient care. Now that the distribution infrastructure and processes have been worked out for nighttime coverage, NightHawk and its successor vRad and some of the other, larger nighttime providers are using the same teleradiology systems to enable fellowship-trained radiologists to provide daytime subspecialty readings.

In his 2007 American College of Radiology (ACR) presidential oration,[13] Jim Borgstede warned about letting technologies such as teleradiology control us instead of vice versa He warned about commoditization and the savaging of radiology as a profession. He spoke of the importance of use management, technical supervision, and consultation as the foundation of maintaining our professional stature. This article addresses each of these points in turn in the context of off-site teleradiology.

Although I agree that use management is important for patient safety and for controlling health care costs, we are rarely consulted even in the hospital for most cross-sectional studies; they are simply ordered. Questioning a referring physician's order too often may result in a loss of referrals. We would like to offer the clinicians a (reimbursed) radiology consult, similar to a cardiology consult. This consult would allow us to choose the least expensive, least invasive, and most informative/appropriate test for the patient. However, this radiology consultation does not currently exist (with the possible exception of interventional radiology), although it might be introduced if accountable care organizations (ACOs) become established. In addition, hospitals are becoming increasingly interested in implementing online clinical decision support (CDS) as a way to automatically filter out inappropriate examinations[14] and to forestall implementation of radiology benefits managers for all cases. These systems are generally based on the ACR Appropriateness Criteria bolstered by additional clinical experience from Massachusetts General Hospital (in the case

of Commissure/Nuance) or the Brigham and Women's Hospital (in the case of Medicalis).

Technical supervision can be done as easily for CT or MR imaging from off site as in the hospital. When I first started providing MR imaging overreads in February 1984, part of the service was protocoling of the next day's cases and image quality assessment. Although the films arrived by overnight courier rather than by teleradiology at that time, the technical supervision was still being provided from off site. Even today at UCSD, we conduct MR imaging at 5 separate locations, but the MR fellows and subspecialty faculty are generally only physically present at 1 or 2 of them. Thus, protocoling is provided by fax or online from central, subspecialized MR reading areas and image quality assessment is accomplished by reading from PACS and by calling the local technologist, both of which can be accomplished as easily off site as on. It may not always be contemporaneous (as in checking the case before the patient gets off the scanner table), but it could be.

Regarding off-site teleradiology having an impact on consultation, radiologists can interact as easily by phone locally as from off site. Whether on site or off, radiologists are serving as the (frequently unsung) consultant for the patient's best interest. For example, if a clinician orders gadolinium-enhanced MR imaging on a patient on dialysis, it is the radiologist's responsibility to inform both the clinician and the patient about the possibility of developing nephrogenic systemic fibrosis.[15] Radiologists can do this as easily from off site as from the hospital because it is likely to involve a phone call in either case.

In an increasingly busy world in which referring physicians may not have time to leave their patients to take calls, companies like Vocada/Nuance now allow radiologists to contact them with important findings asynchronously (eg, using e-mail). When a wet reading is requested or an unexpected finding found, the referring physician can be paged and instructed to call a toll-free number for the reading, which is kept as a digitally-tagged voice file, should a medicolegal scenario subsequently arise. Again, this can be done as easily from off site as from on site.

PACS and the Internet have already fundamentally changed how radiology is practiced. It is already giving small and rural radiology practices (an ACR commission previously chaired by Jim Borgstede) access to subspecialty interpretations. Small radiology groups without fellowship-trained subspecialists can now contract out for subspecialty interpretations from local universities or will need to be melded into larger groups to provide this higher level of service that is being increasingly demanded by subspecialty clinicians.

Although there may an element of commoditization in these scenarios, they are improving patient care. In addition, other specialties are becoming similarly commoditized for improved patient care. Take the hospitalists, for example. Until a decade or so ago, internists saw patients in their clinics and followed them when they were admitted to the hospital. Now the hospitalists tend to follow patients in the hospital and the internist may only see the patient in the clinic.

Fifty years ago, radiologists were still striving for recognition as fully-fledged physicians.[1] Once a group was awarded a hospital contract, it was generally theirs forever. Secure that they would always have their hospital contract, some groups began to push the congeniality envelope by (1) installing outpatient MR centers in direct competition with the hospital,[16] (2) not showing up for medical staff meetings, and (3) not responding to hospital requests for more subspecialist radiologists, all which clearly annoy the administration. Radiologists also annoy the other medical specialists who are envious of their high salaries and presumed regular hours. Internists and pediatricians who have been up all night are dismayed to see radiologists driving their Porsches and Mercedes (no longer Toyota Celicas) into the doctors' parking lot.[17] All these people need is a small excuse, like a few diagnostic misses or patient complaints, to influence the powers that be to cancel the radiologists' contracts.

Because the digital infrastructure needed for teleradiology can also be used to rapidly staff the diagnostic portion of a radiology department, some of the larger teleradiology companies have taken over local hospital contracts. By having a few radiologists on the ground for consults, committees, and procedures, the rest of the studies can be sent out by teleradiology to subspecialists. Some might argue that this is better patient care, particularly if the displaced group only had general radiologists. When this change is driven by the teleradiology companies, it is viewed as predatory.[16] When there were 2 publicly traded teleradiology companies (NightHawk and Virtual Radiology), it could have been argued that the companies needed to be more responsive to their shareholders than to their patients. With ~80 teleradiology companies vying for the limited nighttime business, competition has lowered their charges per read, forcing the public companies into daytime subspecialty reads that might include taking over hospital contracts. However, when NightHawk and Virtual Radiology were both acquired by Provident and relabeled vRad, they ceased being public companies. Regardless, radiology groups should strive to

become even more helpful to the clinicians and administrators in this new environment because it is easy for us to be replaced.[18]

Many of the factors discussed earlier depend on whether there is a shortage or surfeit of radiologists. When NightHawk came into being during the past decade, there was a shortage of radiologists, and emergency CT studies performed at night were rapidly increasing.[9] There was no way a radiologist could be up all night and then work the next day. Giving the radiologist the next day off was a luxury only the larger groups could afford and, even then, it was a sizable expense. Smaller groups that tried to insource nighttime reads found that they were paying top dollar for only reading a limited number of studies (ie, the nighttime radiologist was not adequately loaded). NightHawk afforded the economies of scale by having fully loaded radiologists at night whose work was facilitated by local helpers and digital aids such as voice recognition. Thus the cost of contracting with NightHawk was less than insourcing the same work. In addition, groups with nighttime teleradiology coverage were better at attracting young radiologists with family commitments in a competitive market, so it is easy to see why NightHawk was so successful. However, at the time of this writing, there is no longer such a shortage of radiologists. Recently trained radiologists now take any job they can get, even if it means taking night call.

SUMMARY

PACS and the Internet have changed how clinicians interact with their clinical colleagues, both during the day and at night. Teleradiology may improve the quality of life for radiologists but it also improves the quality of the interpretations for the patients, particularly if the radiologist is a subspecialist reading during the daytime. Given the opportunity this provides to connect subspecialist clinicians with subspecialist radiologists, daytime and nighttime teleradiology is likely to increase. Although teleradiology may worsen the commoditization that started with PACS, patient care will likely be improved, and that should always be the highest priority.

REFERENCES

1. Maynard CD. Radiologists: physicians or expert image interpreters? Radiology 2008;248:333–6.
2. Bradley WG. Off-site radiology: the pros. Radiology 2008;248:337–41.
3. Hawk P. Teleradiology: friend or foe? What imaging's now indispensable partner means for radiology's

future and for the quality of care. J Health Care Finance 2011;37(4):71–92.

4. Medicare's reimbursement for interpretations of hospital emergency room x-rays. U.S. Department of Health and Human Services, Office of the Inspector General; 1993. Available at: http://oig.hhs.gov/oei/reports/oei-02-89-01490.pdf. Accessed January 5, 2012.

5. D'Agincourt L. Best of teleradiology: how it's being done. Diagn Imaging (San Franc) 1994;16(4):41, 45–51.

6. Wilson AJ. Is teleradiology the solution to after-hours emergency radiology coverage? Radiographics 1996;16(4):939–42.

7. Franken EA. Teleradiology moving into the mainstream. Telemed Today 1996;4(1):14–5.

8. DeCorato DR, Kagestu NJ, Ablow RC. Off-hours interpretation of radiologic images of patients admitted to the emergency room department: efficacy of teleradiology. Am J Roentgenol 1995;165(5):1293–6.

9. Bradley WG. Offshore teleradiology. J Am Coll Radiol 2004;1(4):244–8.

10. Social Security Act. § 1862(a)(4). 42 USC § 1395y(a)(4).

11. Bradley WG. Use of a nighthawk service in an academic radiology department. J Am Coll Radiol 2007;4(10):675–7.

12. Lewis RS, Sunshine JH, Bhargavan M. Radiology practices' use of external off-hours teleradiology services in 2007 and changes since 2003. Am J Roentgenol 2009 Nov;193(5):1333–9.

13. Borgstede JP. 2007 ACR presidential oration: four foundations for our future. J Am Coll Radiol 2007;4:875–8.

14. Sistrom CL, Dang PA, Weilburg JB, et al. Effect of computerized order entry with integrated decision support on the growth of outpatient procedure volumes: seven-year time series analysis. Radiology 2009;251(1):147–55 [Epub 2009 Feb 12].

15. Kanal E, Barkovich AJ, Bell C, et al. ACR blue ribbon panel on MR safety. ACR guidance document for safe MR practices: 2007. AJR Am J Roentgenol 2007; 188(6):1447–74.

16. Levin DC, Rao VM. Outsourcing to teleradiology companies: bad for radiology, bad for radiologists. J Am Coll Radiol 2011;8(2):104–8.

17. Mallon W. Available at: http://www.epmonthly.com/columns/in-my-opinion/the-life-cycle-of-a-parasitic-specialist/. Accessed January 5, 2012.

18. Rao VM, Levin DC. The value-added services of hospital-based radiology groups. J Am Coll Radiol 2011;8(9):626–30.

Conflict of Interest in Neuroradiology

Patrick A. Turski, MD

KEYWORDS

• Conflict of interest • Significant financial interest • Commercial interest • Management plan

KEY POINTS

- Federal guidelines require that human subjects investigators report all outside activities greater than $5000 in value to their institutional conflict of interest committee.
- Conflicts of interest in practice occur when a financial interest may influence clinical decision making.
- Educational programs can be compromised by financial conflicts of interest and appropriate disclosure is required before presentations.

INTRODUCTION

Patients need to feel confident that the decisions made by the physicians caring for them are not influenced by personal financial interests. Pharmaceutical companies and medical imaging equipment manufacturers are examples of entities that have the potential to influence the decision making of Neuroradiologists. When significant financial involvement with industry occurs, the activity must be disclosed to the Institution's conflict of interest committee or adminitrative personnel. It is important to note that some interactions with industry can have a positive impact on patient care by accelerating the introduction of new technologies.[1] However, the pervasiveness of these relationships has generated public concern that financial interests may adversely impact clinical managment. Federal agencies,[2] Legal Actions[3] Academic Organizations[4] and Professional Institutes[5] have all brought into focus the potential of financial interest to compromise clinical judgment. The Institute of Medicine report[5] describes a conflict of interest (COI) as a set of circumstances that creates a risk that professional judgment or actions regarding the care of a patient will be unduly influenced by a secondary interest. An individual COI occurs when a person with entrusted responsibility (eg, patient care, education, research) has another interest that may conflict with the proper exercise of that responsibility.

Radiologists have a broad range of experiences in many aspects of health care. These qualities are of value to industry, and neuroradiologists are often invited to participate in clinical advisory groups or provide consultation to industry regarding product development. The presence of outside interests, and the COIs that may result, are not completely avoidable. However, even the perception of COI undermines public trust and patients may become concerned about the safety of new imaging techniques and treatments. It is imperative that physicians address COIs to maintain the public trust, which can be accomplished by

Disclosure: The University of Wisconsin, Department of Radiology, receives research support from GE Healthcare, Waukesha, Wisconsin. A portion of this support is budgeted for research personnel under the direction of Dr Patrick Turski. Dr Turski also serves as Principal Investigator for NIH RO1NS066982. He has an equity interest in Ultrasonix, a privately held device manufacturer of diagnostic ultrasound equipment and Novelos Therapeutics, a biotechnology company.
Division of Neuroradiology, University of Wisconsin School of Medicine and Public Health, 600 Highland Avenue, Madison, WI 53792-3252, USA
E-mail address: pturski@uwhealth.org

reporting all significant financial interests, developing management plans when COIs occur, and disclosing financial conflict to the public. There are many aspects of COI, but this article focuses on financial COIs in human subject research, neuroradiology practice, and education.

MILESTONES IN COI

The Bayh-Dole Act of 1980, also called the Patent and Trademark Amendment and the Stevenson-Wydler Technology Innovation Act, promote university-industrial interactions by allowing researchers and universities to retain ownership of intellectual property resulting from federally funded research and to license the discoveries to industry. This highly successful legislation greatly accelerates the transition of research innovations into commercial products. Relationships between physicians and industry start to proliferate.[1]

The Public Health Service report released in 1995 (PHS; 60 FR 35815, 42 CFR 50) outlines the responsibilities of federal grant applicants regarding financial COI. The goal is to promote objectivity, honesty, and integrity in research. Initial compliance with the regulations is variable and there is no uniform approach across institutions.[2]

A landmark case occurs in 1999, when Jesse Gelsinger dies following a gene transfer experiment. Controversy ensues when it was revealed that the principal investigator and his university had major ownership interests in the company providing the gene transfer product. The concept of financial COI was brought into the public debate. Research institutions aggressively move to establish guidelines for monitoring and managing COI in research.[3]

In 2007 the Association of American Medical Colleges and the Association of American Universities issue a joint report and revised COI guidelines. The report provides a framework for all academic institutions to meet the recommended COI standards, and templates are made available for local COI committees.[4]

In 2009 the Institute of Medicine publishes a comprehensive report on "Conflict of Interest in Medical Research, Education and Practice". The report is reviewed by congressional committees and recommendations are made to the US PHS and the Department of Health and Human Services (HHS).[5]

PHS and HHS release the "Final Rule" in 2011 and new regulations regarding financial COI are established for research sponsored by the National Institutes of Health (NIH) and other federal agencies.[6]

In 2012, The Patient Protection and Affordable Health Care Act (H.R. 3590), includes the Physician Payment Sunshine Act, which requires pharmaceutical, medical device, biologic, and medical supply manufacturers to report to the HHS any payment or other transfer of value to physicians and teaching hospitals.[7]

COI IN HUMAN SUBJECTS RESEARCH

Recently, the Public Health Service in collaboration with HHS published in the Federal Register revised financial COI regulations under the heading "Responsibility of Applicants for Promoting Objectivity in Research for which PHS Funding is Sought" (2011PHS/HHS Final Rule).[6] This material supplements the previous regulations published in 1995.[2] The regulations promote standards that ensure that the design, conduct, and reporting of NIH-sponsored research is free of bias from financial COI.

For federally funded research, all investigators must comply with the PHS/HHS guidelines. The 2011PHS/HHS Final Rule clarifies that the term investigator includes the principal investigator and any other person, regardless of title or position, who is responsible for the design, conduct, or reporting of NIH-sponsored research, which includes collaborators and consultants even if they are not receiving salary support from the award. The 2011PHS/HHS Final Rule focuses predominantly on the issue of financial COI. The first requirement is that the research institution establishes an internal system for physicians to annually report all outside activities. The outside activities include financial interests (eg, remuneration, stock, stock options, consulting, royalties), leadership roles in industry (eg, officer in a company or member of the board), or ownership in a company. The outside activities report is typically reviewed by an institutional officer and reports indicating potential conflicts are forwarded to the institution's local COI committee.

The institutional COI committee is charged with the task of reviewing the outside activities and determining whether a significant financial interest exists. A significant financial interest of the investigator (or of the investigator's spouse and dependent children) is described in the 2011PHS/HHS Final Rule as arising when, for a publicly traded entity, the value of any remuneration or equity interest (eg, stock or stock options) received from the entity in the 12 months preceding the disclosure exceeds $5000. For non–publicly traded entities, a significant financial interest exists if the value of the remuneration exceeds $5000 or when the investigator holds any equity interest, stock, stock options, patent license fees (if paid directly to the investigator), ownership interest, or leadership position (eg, paid officer of the company). Investigators are also required to disclose sponsored travel expenses (see **Box 1**). The regulations also require that the COI reports are made available to the public, either by posting on a Web site or by providing a mechanism for written requests. The 201PHS/HHS Final Rule reiterates that a financial COI exists when the financial conditions could directly and significantly affect the design, conduct, or reporting of NIH-funded research.

Most institutional COI committees use a financial threshold (either as an arbitrarily defined amount or as a percentage of income) to define significant financial interest. Other potential conflicts such as leadership or ownership in a commercial entity are also evaluated. If the financial threshold is

exceeded or there is leadership/ownership in the entity and a nexus is present between the proposed research and the financial interest, the physician is not allowed to proceed with the research. If the financial threshold is exceeded or there is leadership/ownership in the entity but there is no nexus with the proposed research, the investigator may be allowed to proceed with the research with a management plan approved by the institutional COI committee. There is some variability across institutions in the financial threshold that requires management, with reported thresholds ranging from $5000 to $10,000. The relevant information from the internal COI committee review is then disclosed to the funding agency (eg, NIH). The major elements of the process are summarized in **Fig. 1**.

The following example is how the process works at one institution. During a low point in the stock

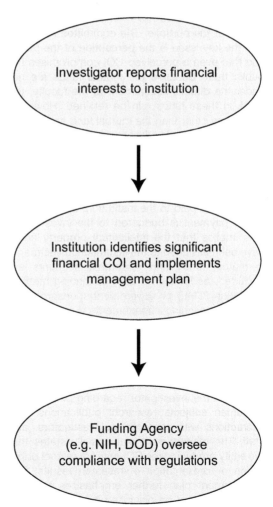

Fig. 1. Framework for oversight of financial COI in research. DOD, Department of Defense.

market, a neuroradiology faculty member decides to invest in several publicly traded companies thought to be undervalued. One of the stocks selected is a multinational company (company A) of which 1 division manufactures medical imaging equipment. The faculty member updates his outside activities report to indicate new investments that exceed the institution's threshold. The report is reviewed by staff and forwarded to the institution COI committee. The committee review notes that the faculty member is part of a research group that receives support from a division of company A. Because the faculty member's research involves human subjects, the committee disqualifies the faculty member from participating in the research because of a financial COI and notifies the local Institutional review board. The faculty member responds to the committee indicating that, because of the size of company A, any activities in his research domain could have no meaningful impact on the stock value; several of his mutual funds have similar stock holdings as part of the portfolio. The committee responds that the key issue is the perception of the public and that even a perceived COI compromises the public trust. Because the mutual funds are not under the direct management of the faculty, the stock in these funds can be retained. However, the shares other than the mutual fund are directly managed by the faculty member and therefore represent a financial COI. The faculty member was required to divest the stock before resuming participation in the human subjects protocol.

COI exclusions include royalties and license fees that are paid to the institution, and a portion of the payment is budgeted to the investigator. This implies that the intellectual property rights have been assigned to the institution. Investments in mutual funds and retirement accounts are excluded, as is income from continuing medical education (CME) or government-sponsored lectures and teaching engagements. For additional details, the HHS/NIH has a Web site that contains a comprehensive archive and summarizes relevant federal regulations.[8]

Management plans for investigators with financial COIs describe the requirements that are placed on the investigator regarding participation in human subjects research, publications, and interactions with students, coinvestigators, and staff. The management plan usually states that the entity producing the COI may not restrict publication or presentation of research results. The management plan further emphasizes that the relationship must be disclosed in all publications and presentations. The form of the disclosure should conform to established recommendations of the journal or the education program and be similar to the following examples: Dr A has an ownership interest in company 1, which has licensed the technology reported in this publication or the research reported was supported by funding provided by company 1, in which Dr A has a significant financial interest.

Federal regulations state that the institution has a responsibility to ensure that COIs do not negatively affect students, residents, fellows, coinvestigators, or research staff. The COI committee usually requires, via the management plan, that the investigator inform all students, residents, fellows, coinvestigators, and research staff of the COI in a written statement that explains the relationship with the entity and emphasizes the right of the individual to bring any concerns to the attention of the Dean, Director, or COI committee. The communication should include a description of the investigator's role in the company, the purpose of the company, the relationship to the investigator's work, restrictions placed on the work, and ownership of intellectual property connected to the company. The document should be signed by both parties.

In most instances, an investigator cannot participate in a human subjects protocol if the investigator has a significant financial interest in an entity that sponsors the study or if the investigator owns or licenses a technology tested in the study. Exceptions are occasionally granted by the institutional COI committee if the research cannot be conducted safely and effectively without the individual. If an exception is granted, other restrictions may be applied, such as monitoring of research by independent peers, modification of the research plan, or disqualification from participation in a portion of the research. In some situations, severance of the relationship, including divestiture of the financial interest, may be the only option to allow participation in the human subjects protocol.

The purpose of the Physician Payment Sunshine Act is to increase the transparency of the relationship between vendors and physicians. The Physician Payment Sunshine Act is part of the Patient Protection and Affordable Healthcare Act (H.R. 3590) and requires pharmaceutical, medical device, biologic, and medical supply manufacturers to report to HHS any payment or other transfer of value to physicians and teaching hospitals. The first reports are due March 31, 2013, for the calendar year 2012 reporting period. The reports will include the amount of the payment, date, and the nature of the payment. Gifts, consulting fees, and entertainment will be included in the reports. The Physician Payment Sunshine Act will preempt any state disclosure laws that cover similar activities. The information will be available to the public at request. It is unclear at this point how the information will be managed by HHS.

The Physician Payment Sunshine Act excludes certain types of payments from its disclosure requirements. Manufacturers are not required to disclose information concerning the following types of payments: (1) transfer of anything the value of which is less than $10, (2) product samples, (3) educational materials, (4) the loan of a medical device for a short-term trial period, (5) discounts, (6) in-kind items used for the provision of charity care, or (7) a dividend or other profit distribution from a publicly traded mutual fund.

COI IN PRACTICE

Physicians are required to maintain the highest level of professionalism, and many institutions have developed detailed policies to oversee the interactions of physicians with industry.[9] The University of Wisconsin (UW) Medical Foundation policy is used as an example in this article of how one institution manages this issue.[10]

In the UW policy, providers are not allowed to accept gifts from industry. There is no minimum value and even gifts as small as pens, note pads, and laser pointers are not allowed. Gifts of money, property, service, food, travel, and entertainment are strictly prohibited. Nonbranded, nonpromotional patient education materials may be accepted under the oversight of the institution provided that the materials are not gifted on behalf of an individual faculty member.

All physicians are required to report outside financial relationships with industry on an annual basis. In the report, the faculty member lists each company for which a relationship exists, a description of the type of activity, remuneration received, and whether educational activities were approved by the American Academy for Continuing Medical Education. Disclosure to patients is accomplished by listing the reports on a Web site and posting notifications in the various clinics indicating that some providers have financial interests with industry. Patients are invited to contact the institution for specific information about their clinician.

Attendance at events that are funded by industry but not certified by the CME is acceptable as long as physicians pay all of their own expenses. The physician cannot receive any payment or gifts for attending the event, including the cost of the meal, travel, or accommodations. The UW policy prohibits the participation of physicians in speaker's bureaus, contracted educational programs, or other non-CME programs that are promotional and funded by pharmaceutical or biologic industry. One exception to this rule is the participation of physicians in non-CME events sponsored by device manufacturers if training in the device is required by the US Food and Drug Administration (FDA).[11] Participation in vendor-sponsored device training is subject to the US Department of Justice September 2007 deferred prosecution agreements, which include (1) fair market compensation not to exceed $500 per hour, (2) management plan for notice to and interaction with patients, (3) written contract establishing clear deliverables, and (4) reasonable reimbursement for lodging, travel, and dining expenses.[12] At UW, the physician must also submit the presentation and/or device training program for approval from an independent committee (the UW Industry Interaction Review Committee), which then grants permission for the faculty to participate in the event. UW physicians can also petition the UW Industry Interaction Review Committee to allow the faculty member to participate in non-CME events that are unique international learning opportunities.

In general, consultation with industry is an accepted activity for UW physicians. The typical activities include expert consultation, serving on advisory boards, serving as medical directors, and serving on data safety and monitoring boards for clinical trials. The compensation is not to exceed $500 per hour. At UW, the physicians must submit their consulting agreements for review to ensure that there is no conflict with patient care and that the deliverables are clearly defined at fair market value. Providers may own equity in, or serve in, leadership roles for industry under the supervision of the COI committee and after a management plan has been developed for interactions with patients. Royalties from sales of commercial products (eg, new endovascular devices) are permissible as long as there are no payments for sales at UW, that the provider discloses this to the patient, and that the monetary value of the royalty payment is reported annually. A management plan for interactions with patients is always required when royalty payments are linked to clinical care.

Pharmaceutical representatives may meet with physicians but only in a nonclinical space. The appointments with physicians and promotional activities must be approved and overseen by the vendor liaison office. With advanced notice, medical device representatives may enter patient care areas when the visit is requested by the physician and the visit is of direct benefit to the patient.

All industry-sponsored scholarships and other educational funds for trainees must be donated freely (no quid pro quo) to the institution or the department and publicly disclosed. The selection of individuals for scholarships and fellowships must occur independently of the donor and is the responsibility of the training program director or the institution. Pharmaceutical samples, such as complementary vials of contrast medium, cannot be made on behalf of an individual physician.[13] UW physicians are not allowed to participate in publications (or use slides) that have been written by industry. In addition, all costs related to purchasing decisions must be covered by the institution, not by the vendor.

COI IN EDUCATION

The Accreditation Council for Continuing Medical Education (ACCME) has established standards to ensure the independence of CME programs.[14] The standards address independence, personal COIs, commercial support, management of commercial promotion, elimination of commercial bias, and disclosures.

CME activities must be independent of commercial interest, specifically excluding any influence by a vendor that produces, markets, distributes, or profits from the sale of health care goods or services.

The CME course organizers are required to show that participants have disclosed all relevant financial interests of any amount occurring within the prior 12 months that creates a potential COI.

When commercial support is involved, the course organizers must make all decisions regarding the content of the course. All management of financial activities shall be independent of the vendor and used for travel, lodging, honoraria, or personal expenses for bona fide employees and volunteers of the course, joint academic sponsor, or educational partner. A written agreement is required that defines the conditions and purpose of the commercial support.

Management of commercial promotion such as commercial exhibits or advertisements is the responsibility of the course directors. The commercial activities cannot interfere with the CME programming. There can be no juxtaposition of advertising and educational material. The source of all support from commercial interests shall be disclosed to the participants.

The content of the course should provide a balanced review of the topic. The goal is to promote improvement in health care, and promotion of a commercial interest is to be avoided.

Anyone with control over the CME content in the course is required to disclose any relevant commercial relationship, including the name and

nature of the relationship. The disclosure should be made before the beginning of the educational activity. The complete description of the policy can be found on the ACCME Web site.[14]

INSTITUTIONAL COI

Institutional financial COIs can develop when the institution, the senior management or trustees, a department, school, or other subunit has an external financial interest in a company that itself has a financial interest in a faculty research project.[5] Conflicts may also arise when leaders of the institution also serve on boards of companies that have a commercial transaction with the institution. Even the perception of a conflict can lead to suspicion and loss of public trust. The leaders of the institution are best served by comprehensively reporting all of their significant financial interests. After reporting, a management plan can be put into place that reduces the risks to the individual and institution. When necessary, activities should be prohibited to protect the public interest or institution. The key action is to separate the decision making from the financial and research activities so that they can be independently managed. Institution leaders should foster an atmosphere of openness, accountability, and integrity.[15]

In summary, to maintain the public trust, neuroradiologists should participate in COI programs that encompass reporting, review, management of the conflict, prohibition of the activity when necessary, and disclosure.

REFERENCES

1. Title 37–patents, trademarks, and copyrights –rights. Rights to inventions made by nonprofit organizations and small business firms under government grants, contracts, and cooperative agreements. 2002 37(1) Code of Federal Regulations 401. Available at: http://www.access.gpo.gov/nara/cfr/waisidx_99/37cfr 401_99.htm. Accessed January 10, 2012.
2. Responsibility of applicants for promoting objectivity in research for which PHS funding is sought. Federal Register 1995, 60, 35815, the Code of Federal Regulations Title 42 Volume 1 parts 1–399. Available at: http://grants.nih.gov/grants/compliance/42_ CFR_50_Subpart_F.htm. Accessed December 15, 2011.
3. Fox J. Gene-therapy death prompts broad civil lawsuit. Nat Biotechnol 2000;18:1136.
4. A report of the AAMC-AAU Advisory Committee on Financial Conflicts of Interest in Human Subject Research. Protecting patients, preserving integrity, advancing health: accelerating the implementation

of COI policies in human subject research. 2008. Available at: https://members.aamc.org. Accessed December 15, 2011.

5. Institute of Medicine. Conflict of interest in medical research, education, and practice. Washington, DC: The National Academies Press; 2009. p. 1–414.

6. Responsibility of applicants for promoting objectivity in research for which PHS funding is sought and responsible prospective contractors. Federal Register 2011;76(165):52292–3256. Available at: http://www.gpo.gov/fdsys/pkg/FR-2011-08-25/pdf/2011-21633.pdf. Accessed December 22, 2011.

7. Patient Protection and Affordable Health Care Act (H.R. 3590) signed into law in March 2010 subsection Physician Payment Sunshine Act (section 6002) (PPSA). Federal Register 1999;(64): 25260–70.

8. Financial conflict of interest. US Department of Health and Human Services Office of Extramural Support. Available at: http://grants.nih.gov/grants/policy/coi/. Accessed January 13, 2012.

9. Bennan TA, Rothman DJ, Blank L, et al. Health industry practices that create conflicts of interest: a policy proposal for academic medical centers. JAMA 2006;295(4):429–33.

10. Policy on interactions with industry. University of Wisconsin Medical Foundation; 2011. Available at: http://www2.medicine.wisc.edu/home/files/UWMF_Policy_on_Interactions_with_Industry1.pdf. Accessed January 5, 2011.

11. Code of ethics on interactions with healthcare professionals. Advanced Medical Technology Association (AdvaMed) revised 2009. Available at: http://www.advamed.org/NR/rdonlyres/61D30455-F7E9-4081-B219-12D6CE347585/0/AdvaMedCodeofEthicsRevisedandRestatedEffective20090701.pdf. Accessed January 5, 2012.

12. Synopsis of the deferred prosecution agreements. Available at: http://www.usdoj.gov/opa/pr/2007/November/07_civ_873.html. Accessed January 5, 2012.

13. Code on interactions with healthcare professionals. Available at: http://www.phrma.org/sites/default/files/108/phrma_marketing_code_2008.pdf. Accessed January 5, 2012.

14. ACCME standards for commercial support. Available at: http://www.accme.org/dir_docs/doc_upload/68b2902a-fb73-44d1-8725-80a1504e520c_upload document.pdf. Accessed December 22, 2011.

15. Task Force on Research Accountability. Report on individual and institutional financial conflict of interest. Association of American Universities; 2001. Available at: www.aau.edu/research/COI.01.pdf. Accessed January 5, 2012.

Medicolegal Hazards
Potential Pitfalls for Neuroimagers

Paul E. Kim, MD*, Mark S. Shiroishi, MD

KEYWORDS

- Malpractice • Standard of care • Common law • Negligence • Error • Judgment • Perception
- Communication

KEY POINTS

- There are 4 conditions for malpractice: (1) physician-patient relationship, (2) breach of standard of care, (3) injury to patient, and (4) proximate cause.
- There are 3 forms of error in radiology: (1) errors of perception, (2) errors of cognition, and (3) errors of protocol.
- Failure to diagnose is the most common cause of malpractice against a radiologist.
- However, failure to follow established protocols, such as communicating significant findings, are the least defensible.
- Common areas of litigation in neuroradiology include the following: postoperative infection, missed cervical spine injury, missed dural arteriovenous fistula, venous thrombosis.

"On the television program, Law and Order, a defense lawyer, frustrated in her attempt to plea bargain with the prosecuting attorney, threatened to go to court to get a better deal. She stated, 'It's easier to confuse a jury than convince a judge.'[1] Is that not what a plaintiff's attorney relies on in a medical malpractice suit? Confuse the jury. Win the 'lottery'. Many of us think that juries cannot understand the complex medical issues, yet some will grant both deserving and undeserving plaintiffs astronomic awards, providing the attorneys obscene fees. In other cases, truly injured plaintiffs may not get compensated."[1]

INTRODUCTION

In Germany, the United Kingdom, and most Canadian provinces, malpractice judgments are decided by a judge; the United States is one of the few countries in which a jury determines whether a physician has committed malpractice. Sweden and New Zealand have no-fault systems.[2]

"History records that the money changers have used every form of abuse, intrigue, deceit, and violent means possible to maintain their control..."[3]

—James Madison

Although Madison's comments were specifically meant in reference to central banking, the

Financial disclosures: Dr. Shiroishi is supported in part by the GE Healthcare/RSNA Research Scholar Grant.
Department of Radiology, University of Southern California Keck School of Medicine, 1200 North State Street, Room 3740, Los Angeles, CA 90033, USA
* Corresponding author.
E-mail address: pek@usc.edu

sentiment that money changers, today constituted of the banking and insurance industries, have been an iniquitous force in society has been universally held for millennia. In 1957, malpractice insurance rates were between $64 per year and $106 per year in New York and between $300 and $400 per year in California.[4] Today, the average premium paid by neurosurgeons across the country is more than $100,000, with rates more than $300,000 in some states.[5]

According to the California Department of Insurance, medical malpractice insurance rates may be too high because some insurers are spending as little as 2% or 3% of premiums to pay out claims. Insurers in California spent an average of 23% of collected premiums on claims and other losses. California's largest malpractice insurer, The Doctors Company, spent only 10% of the $179 million collected in premiums on claims in 2009.[6] According to Tillinghast, an actuarial consultancy, from 1975 to 2003, the cost of medical malpractice lawsuits increased more than 2000% to $26.5 billion.[7] In 1984, the total federal cost of medical malpractice in the United States, including the costs of the practice of defensive medicine and direct litigation costs, such as malpractice premiums and defending claims, was estimated at $12.1 billion to $13.7 billion, which was approximately 15% of the total physician expenditures that year.[7] By 1991, the inflation-adjusted figure was estimated at $24.9 billion in total liability and system costs.[8] In 2008, overall annual medical liability system costs, including defensive medicine, were estimated to be $55.6 billion or 2.4% of total health care spending. Most of the cost, an estimated $45.6 billion, was caused by defensive medicine, including tests or treatments performed largely to avoid potential lawsuits.[9]

Statistics for the risk of being sued for neuroradiology as a specific subspecialty are unknown, but Jena and colleagues[10] found, in a study published recently in the New England Journal of Medicine, that diagnostic radiology ranked 18th among 25 medical specialties based on the risk of being sued for malpractice, at 7.2% per year versus the overall average of 7.4% of all physicians, with lower-than-average payouts. The fact that this rate is low compared with other medical specialties, and probably less than the risk perceived by radiologists themselves,[11] is little consolation to those who have been involved as a defendant in this process. The risk of being sued at some point in one's radiology career is extremely high, although official statistics seem lower.[12] The authors do not know any radiologists who have been in practice for more than 15 years who have

not experienced a malpractice claim as a defendant. Although most cases result in settlement before trial, only 1% of cases that do go on to trial result in judgments for the plaintiffs. Of the cases that go to trial, physicians are found to be not negligent 83% of the time, yet the physician still loses: first because defense costs (not including decreased productivity related to physician time spent in litigation activities, which can be significant) now average more than $94,000 per case[13] and second because for most physicians the experience of being sued is so traumatic that, although difficult to quantify, it exacts a significant toll on their mental and physical health.[14]

Because some basic understanding of the medicolegal litigation process is essential to adopt effective strategies in avoiding lawsuits, a brief review of the process of medical malpractice litigation follows, including a narrative of the evolution of legal definitions of malpractice. It is hoped that this will provide practical information as to the common pitfalls of medical malpractice from the authors' perspective as neuroradiologists who are not legal experts but who have some experience in malpractice litigation both as defendants and expert witnesses.

HOW WE GOT HERE: DEVELOPMENT OF THE CONCEPTS AND DEFINITIONS OF MEDICAL MALPRACTICE TORT

There are 3 sources of law in the United States: constitutional law revolves around federal and state constitutions; statutory law regards federal and state regulations enacted by government legislatures; and common law, based on the principle of stare decisis (let the decision stand), in which judicial decisions serve as precedents for future decisions made by courts. This is distinguished from civil law, in which all judicial decisions are based on interpretation of applicable statutes rather than precedents of prior court decisions. Common law had its origins in medieval England, and medical malpractice falls under this rubric. In 1765, British legal scholar Sir William Blackstone in his book, Commentaries on the Laws of England, referred to the "neglect or unskillful management of a physician or surgeon" as "mala praxis,"[15] from which the modern term malpractice is derived. The first recorded malpractice case in the United States occurred in 1794.[16]

The modern concept of a standard of care to which physicians may be held liable was not established until 1769 in the case of Slater v Baker and Stapleton.[17] At the time, as hard as it may be to fathom, physician liability may not have been limited to breaching a standard established by other professionals, so the decision in this case had the effect of shielding physicians from most of the tort claims at the time. The court ruled that a physician could be found liable only if another physician testified that a breach of the standard of care had occurred. Additionally, the court required that the expert witness must come from the defendant's own locality, thus establishing the principle of a community standard.

One of the earliest state supreme court decisions regarding medicolegal standard of care was an 1832 case of a patient who had successfully sued a physician in a lower court for pain and irreparable harm after making an incision into her arm to instill the smallpox vaccine. The defendant physician appealed the case to the Connecticut Supreme Court, arguing that because physicians cannot warranty their work or guarantee an outcome, only gross ignorance or gross negligence can subject the physician to damages. The court did not accept this argument and found in favor of the plaintiff (patient), but with significant qualifiers. In an eloquent statement, the court articulated the difficult balancing act between true negligence and perfect outcomes courts must perform in determining the standard of care in any given case[18]:

> *What man, even of skill and talent, would undertake to practice in the healing art, if some little failure of ordinary skill or ordinary diligence, or even some trifling want of carefulness, might sweep from him the whole earnings of a life of toil and drudgery? Restricted to the narrow ground of the charge, many skillful and able physicians would not escape liability a single year of their practice. "Ordinary" means usual, common. The difference between a want of ordinary or useful skill and gross negligence is essential and important. If you were to draw a line of distinction just halfway between the eminently learned physicians and those grossly ignorant, would you not hit exactly on those styled ordinary?...To say that a physician did not perform a certain operation with ordinary skill conveys a very different idea from the assertion that he performs it with gross negligence.*[18]

Such was the origin of the legal concept of ordinary skill and diligence as the appropriate measure of the standard of care rather than the polar extremes of perfect outcome and gross negligence. In 1853, the pendulum swung in the opposite direction, helping to relieve physicians of the

burden of what would in essence be a warranty for work done. The Pennsylvania Supreme Court reversed a lower court's decision finding that a physician had been negligent in setting a comminuted fracture of the tibia and fibula resulting in deformity and limb-length discrepancy.[19]

> *The question is not whether the doctor had brought to the case skill enough to make the leg as straight and long as the other, but whether he had employed such skill and diligence as are ordinarily exercised in his profession. For less than this he is responsible in damages, but if he be held to the measure laid down by the trial court, the implied contract amounts on his part to a warranty of cure for which there is no authority in law.*[19]

There is obviously a vast domain of distinguishing factors and nuance lying between the extremes of gross negligence and perfect outcome, and it is within this vast domain that the standard of care lays. This battleground is the one on which medical malpractice litigation proceeds on a daily basis (**Fig. 1**). Several other decisions were rendered in the mid to late nineteenth century that essentially echoed the sentiments of the Pennsylvania Supreme Court.[2] An important nuance to be explored in this context arose from a New York Supreme Court decision in 1905 in which a crucial legal separation was made between judgment error versus negligence.[20]

> *The law requires a physician to possess the skill and learning which is possessed by the average member of the medical profession... and to apply that skill and learning with ordinary reasonable care. He is not liable for a mere error in judgment, provided he does what he thinks is best after a careful examination. He does not guarantee a good result.*[20]

MALPRACTICE AND THE RADIOLOGIST

Common to all of the historical higher court decisions are the words, *reasonable*, *ordinary*, and *average*, in describing what constitutes the standard of care; legal parsing of these terms continues today as an ever-unfinished, ongoing

Gross Negligence . ? . ? . ? . ? Standard of care? . ? . ? . ? . ? . Perfect Outcome

Fig. 1. Scales of justice in medical malpractice. Medical malpractice case law, particularly since the nineteenth century, has been a balancing act of finding the equitable point of reconciliation between the extremes of gross negligence and perfect outcome in defining liability. Where each individual malpractice case appropriately belongs along this scale is argued daily in the court system.

process. The relevance of these concepts to radiology was adjudicated recently in a case that took up the issue of perceptual errors as it uniquely applies to radiology. The defendant radiologist had settled 2 malpractice lawsuits: one for missing a proximal tibial fracture and another for missing a colon carcinoma on a barium examination. As a result, the Wisconsin Department of Regulation and Licensing subsequently sought to suspend the radiologist's license for conduct it considered negligent but was rebuffed in a lower court, which found in favor of the radiologist. This decision led to an appeal by the department to the state's appellate court, which again found in favor of the radiologist. Crucial to their decision was an analysis of the legal significance of the errors of perception, which are particularly relevant to diagnostic radiology and contain the feared and all too common occurrence of seeing a finding in retrospect. The court's analysis was essentially additional parsing of the recurring concepts of *average* and *reasonable*[21]:

> *"Average physician" is not synonymous with "reasonable physician." The fallacy in the "average" formulation is that it bears no intrinsic relation to what is reasonable….Those that have less than…average skill may still be competent and qualified. Half of the physicians of America do not automatically become negligent in practicing medicine…merely because their skill is less than the professional average. The test is not whether [the radiologist] failed to detect what the average radiologist should have detected, but whether [the defendant radiologist] exercised reasonable care…. [The radiologist] used reasonable and ordinary care, and his failures to detect the abnormalities were "errors in perception."… All radiologists miss abnormalities in X rays, but such errors do not, in and of themselves, constitute negligence in treatment.[21]*

For medical malpractice to have occurred, 4 conditions must be met: (1) there must be a physician-patient relationship, (2) there must have been a breach of the standard of care, (3) the patient must have sustained an injury, and (4) there must be proximate cause (ie, the breach in the standard of care must be the cause of the injury). As has been discussed, making an error does not necessarily mean that the standard of care has been breached. Normal error rates in radiology are typically around 4%[22] to as high as 31% in some studies,[23] but "when is an error simply an error and when is it malpractice?"[24] Legal definitions are meant to be as unambiguous as possible, so the answer to this question requires an analysis of the types of possible errors. Three types of errors are generally encountered: (1) errors of perception, (2) errors of cognition, and (3) errors of protocol.

Errors of perception (ie, missing the finding) constitute 80% of all errors made by radiologists and 70% of radiology malpractice lawsuits, whereas fewer than 30% are cognitive.[25] Here one must distinguish between errors that increase the likelihood of being sued versus the likelihood of losing a lawsuit. Although errors of perception are a frequent cause of malpractice actions being pursued, they are not as likely to result in a *successful* plaintiff's action (ie, judgment against the radiologist). This point is largely because errors in judgment are involved in many cases of perceptual error, and arguments as to the degree of negligence in missing the finding is typically a larger burden for the plaintiff.

The second form of error, errors of cognition, typically occurs when a finding is made but misunderstood, such as calling a normal finding abnormal. It can also occur if a specific entity in a differential diagnosis is not mentioned, either because it was not thought of or because the radiologist did not know. A cognitive error can be the origin of a missed finding when unfamiliarity with a subject directly leads to an inability to perceive or see the finding (**Fig. 2**). Here defensibility resides in establishing a community standard of what is ordinary knowledge versus arcane knowledge and could vary depending on the community (eg, rural vs urban) or practice setting (community vs academic).

The third category of error, protocol errors, is the least defensible. These errors take several forms, including what is by far the most common cause of successful (ie, verdict for the plaintiff) medicolegal action: failure to communicate significant findings. Other errors in this category include permitting a technically inadequate study leading to misdiagnosis, failure to compare prior studies, and failure to make appropriate recommendations. Although these issues are not as commonly

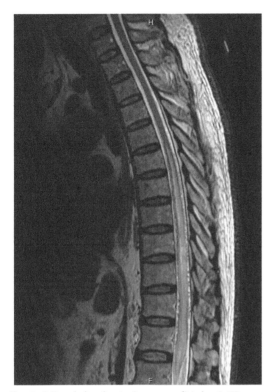

Fig. 2. Missed dural arteriovenous fistula. A 63-year-old male patient with myelopathic signs and MR imaging demonstrating hyperintense signal within the cord on T2-weighted images and multiple small signal voids in the subarachnoid space, which was attributed to normal cerebrospinal fluid pulsation. Because mild gadolinium contrast enhancement was also seen, a spinal cord tumor was suspected and a biopsy was performed.

invoked in lawsuits as failure to communicate, they are nevertheless inherently more difficult to defend because these errors typically result from a failure to follow established and unambiguous standards and guidelines, all of which are delineated by the American College of Radiology.

COMMUNICATION OF IMPORTANT FINDINGS

Although failure to diagnosis is the most common cause of a malpractice action against a radiologist, failure to communicate important findings ranks second, being at least one of the causal factors in 80% of cases.[26] Communication of results may be the most conspicuous action a radiologist can take to reduce litigation risk, yet failure to do so is increasing as a cause of malpractice litigation.[27] That the radiologist bears responsibility for communicating important findings is now almost universally understood, but many radiologists are not well versed as to the full measure of what this duty entails. Actions that some might presume to be

adequate are actually less than the standard of care, with precedents in settled law[28]: (1) relying on the written report to communicate even a nonurgent but unexpected important finding (direct radiologist-to-physician communication, either by telephone or in person, is required[29]); (2) leaving a voicemail; (3) notifying only for urgent findings (unexpected but significant nonurgent findings also require direct notification); (4) making good faith but ultimately unsuccessful attempts to contact a responsible party (in this case, it is also settled law that patients must be contacted and made aware of their condition).[30–32] To the chagrin of most radiologists, opinions written in case law are clearly not sympathetic to the difficulties this may impose on a radiologist in a busy practice, such as in a 1991 case in which a registered nurse was not informed of the possibility of sarcoidosis in a preemployment chest radiograph finding after a negative purified protein derivative (tuberculin) eliminated tuberculosis from the differential diagnosis:

> "We have little trouble holding that the radiologist owed [the plaintiff] a duty... At a minimum, the radiologist should have notified the [the plaintiff] of the abnormality. This duty is hardly burdensome."[31]

Documentation

Failure to document a communication is a major reason why a radiologist will lose a lawsuit even if the communication had diligently occurred. The official report should document the date, time, the person spoken to, and what was said. If a preliminary report is rendered before the final report is prepared, any significant change between the preliminary and final interpretation should be reported directly to the referring physician and that communication should also be documented.[33]

Bias Errors

Bias errors are both perceptual and cognitive in character. There are principally 2 ways in which preconceived notions create errors and both are insidiously common. One way is the absence of relevant clinical information or presence of misleading information. Studies have shown conclusively that the knowledge of clinical history improves radiologic diagnosis,[34,35] and a negative clinical history considerably alters the significance given to a finding in terms of follow-up and management. Elmore and colleagues[36] showed that when a sham clinical history was given, 40% of the radiologists changed their diagnostic interpretation about whether to recommend a biopsy.

The second type of error that bears mentioning in this context is known as the alliterative error. The alliterative error is one in which a prior report influences the interpretation of a current examination. Marcus J. Smith, who coined the term, alliterative error, reasoned that a prior study reported as negative or reported with the wrong significance attached to a finding will increase the likelihood of a subsequent radiologist repeating the error.[37,38] So if one looks at a prior negative report before the imaging study, there is a greater chance of missing a significant abnormality.[38]

COMMON NEUROIMAGING PITFALLS REQUIRING EXTRA CAUTION

The legal principles discussed thus far that are applicable to radiologists (and physicians) also obviously apply to neuroradiologists. The compendium of circumstances more specific to neuroimaging that have resulted in error and ultimately in litigation is rather unwieldy, but there are notable situations in which heightened vigilance is advised because of the frequency that litigation is connected.

The Postoperative State

The postoperative state, whether in the head or spine, creates an especially hazardous condition because of the inherent ambiguity that often exists between normal postoperative findings and dire complications, most frequently infection. Magnetic resonance (MR) imaging findings of diffusion restriction within postoperative blood products (typically extracellular methemoglobin), fluid with surrounding contrast enhancement, dural and leptomeningeal contrast enhancement, and T2 fluid-attenuated inversion recovery (FLAIR) sulcal hyperintensity frequently represent normal postoperative appearances. The same descriptors are also the hallmarks of infection with subdural empyema and meningitis (**Fig. 3**). Especially confounding is that the clinical and even laboratory findings are also frequently unhelpful. Although signs of wound infection are the most common finding, it is sometimes not present; other signs, such as fever and headache, occur in only a minority of patients early in the process, and more than one-third of patients will not have leukocytosis.[39] If leukocytosis is present, it can be erroneously attributed to postoperative steroids administered to decrease brain swelling. In postoperative cases, therefore, caveats as to the nature of expected postoperative findings should be

reported. An increase in the size of a postoperative fluid collection may be the only imaging finding that indicates an abscess and should always be treated as significant. A cautious approach regarding follow-up imaging is also needed, which should be recommended for any significant change in the clinical status of patients.

Missed Cervical Spine Injury

Most malpractice awards for the plaintiff in cases of missed cervical spine (C-spine) injury are *not* fractures[40] but traumatic disk herniations; ligamentous injury; and, probably less commonly, epidural hematomas. Routine computed tomography (CT) scanning of the C-spine in trauma patients is now an accepted convention and has significantly enhanced the detection of fractures and large traumatic disk herniations (**Fig. 4**). Like plain radiography, however, CT lacks sensitivity for the detection of ligamentous injury and instability, thus precipitating the ongoing controversy well known to most radiology departments regarding the use of MR imaging in trauma patients. The reader can refer to a large body of literature on the subject, which remains largely unsettled.[41–44] However, to reduce malpractice risk, one must be generous in recommending MR imaging correlation (**Fig. 5**). MR imaging findings should also be interpreted with caution because MR imaging has a high negative predictive value in the acute phase of C-spine injury and becomes significantly less sensitive after several days because of decreasing edema.[42–44]

Missed Aneurysm

Missing the diagnosis of a cerebral aneurysm of course may have grave consequences for patients and, unfortunately, difficulty in establishing the diagnosis is a frequent occurrence. The false-negative rate of neuroimaging studies is small but not insubstantial, and which imaging modality is best used is not a settled matter.[45,46] Established practice standards or guidelines are generally meant to delineate minimal acceptable practices and have limited medicolegal applicability in these cases and are more relevant when negligence is more straightforward.[47,48] Furthermore, since the advent of MR angiography (MRA) and CT angiography (CTA), the long-established gold standard designation of catheter angiography can no longer be presupposed. There is a true lack of consensus as to whether CTA or catheter angiography is the better test, although it is generally agreed that MRA should be limited for use in the follow-up of cases of unruptured aneurysms when surveillance was elected over surgical or endovascular intervention.[49,50]

A

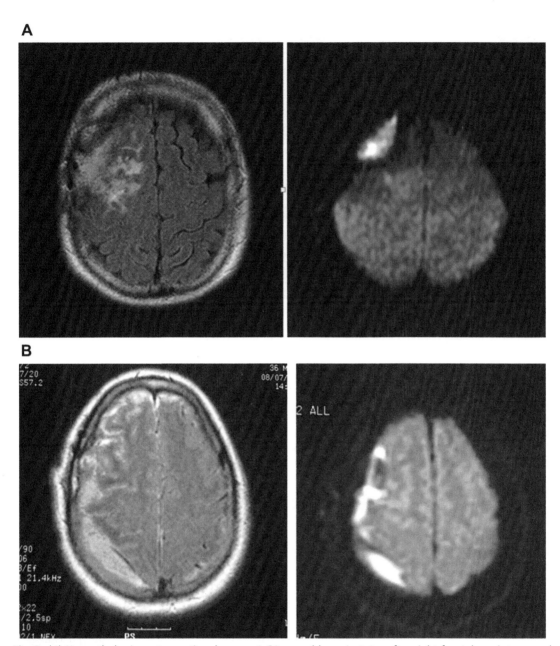

Fig. 3. (A) Nonpathologic postoperative changes. A 64-year-old man's status after right frontal craniotomy and resection of a convexity meningioma. T2 FLAIR (*left*) demonstrates a small mildly hyperintense extra-axial fluid collection over the right frontal convexity and sulcal hyperintensity. Diffusion-weighted trace image (*right*) demonstrates diffusion restriction within the small extracerebral postoperative fluid collection, presumably representing subacute blood products. (B) Postoperative subdural empyema. A 38-year-old man 12 days after meningeal biopsy for abnormal dural thickening and diagnosis of hypertrophic pachymeningitis. The patient presented with a seizure and T2 FLAIR images (*left*) demonstrate mildly hyperintense subdural fluid and sulcal hyperintensity and diffusion restriction within the subdural collection on diffusion-weighted imaging (*right*). Note the similarity to the appearance in (A).

Although the jury is out in the debate over the appropriate gold standard, one should bear in mind that the potentially more hazardous pitfall is likely to be a missed aneurysm diagnosis caused by a faulty angiographic or CTA technique. In fact, although proper technique in catheter angiography is well established and false-negative rates are fairly well defined, standardized CTA methodology is

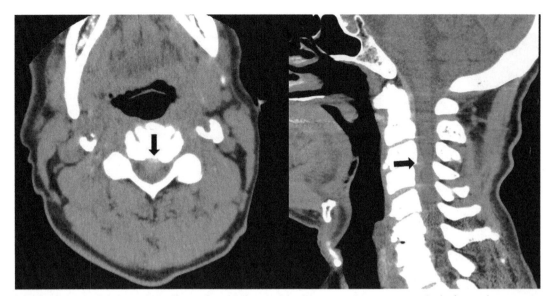

Fig. 4. Traumatic disk herniation (*arrows*). Initially missed when attention was excessively focused on osseous structures resulting in inattention to clearly visible soft tissue findings. The quality of C-spine imaging with current CT technology obligates an adequate assessment of soft tissues.

lacking and varies considerably (particularly in postprocessing methodology); although some investigators note very high sensitivity rivaling or surpassing conventional angiography, the reported sensitivity of CTA for the diagnosis of aneurysms varies widely.[51–55] Differences in postprocessing methodology may be responsible for most of these discrepancies.[56] Thus, because digital subtraction angiography has traditionally been the gold standard, it is incumbent on the radiologist choosing to use CTA that a robust CTA methodology be used. This point is particularly true because it is likely that several aneurysms not initially noted on CTA are present in retrospect.[55]

Other Commonly Missed Pathologic Conditions: More Common in the Non-Neuroradiologist?

The authors note a few additional entities that, in their experience, have more often involved radiologists without formal neuroradiology training, although certainly any neuroradiologist could also be derelict in making these diagnoses: spinal dural arteriovenous fistula (DAVF), dural sinus thrombosis, and thiamine deficiency. In the case of the spinal DAVF, the error is usually of the cognitive type because abnormal vascular flow voids in the spinal subarachnoid space are misinterpreted as normal cerebrospinal fluid pulsations (see **Fig. 2**). Dural sinus thrombosis is simply a difficult diagnosis to make and can be considered one of the holy grails of neuroimaging. Often one must think of the

diagnosis to make it and the findings are frequently subtle.[57]

ADDITIONAL MEDICOLEGAL HAZARDS FOR THE NEUROIMAGER

Two external medicolegal hazards bear mentioning. Statistics are lacking as to the extent negligence on the part of a clinician results in patient injury and a consulting radiologist subsequently being named as a party in a lawsuit but anecdotal observation strongly suggests that this is a significant factor in the risk of being sued. Another issue that defendants and potential defendants must face is the systemic phenomenon of the paid expert witness. Because one side retains them, the expert may act with unconscious bias to further the case of the party they represent. In other cases, experts are unprincipled deliberately. Following the lead of the American Association of Neurologic Surgeons (AANS), which had established an expert witness review program in 1983 and suspended a member for improper expert witness testimony in 2001,[58] the American College of Radiology established a similar review program within its committee on ethics. This formation resulted in the expulsion of a member for the first time in its history in 2004 for improper expert witness testimony.[59] This action had its basis on a landmark ruling by the Seventh Circuit Court of Appeals in a case brought against the AANS by the neurosurgeon they had sanctioned for improper testimony, Donald C. Austin. Dr Austin

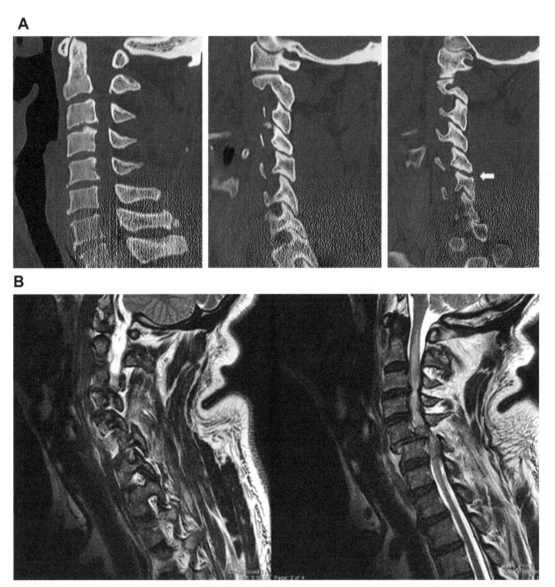

Fig. 5. A 49-year-old man after a severe fall. (A) Initial CT scan was reported as negative for acute posttraumatic findings, with moderate underlying degenerative changes. (B) MR imaging obtained 1 week later when the patient experienced minor trauma and became acutely quadriparetic. Unilateral perched facet is noted on the left image, and severe cord injury caused by unstable 3-column injury is demonstrated on the right. Such cases raise a point of contention regarding what criteria have been used to define normal or negative CT scans in reports studying the necessity of MR imaging for spinal trauma. The initial CT scan showed subtle but definite widening of the right facet joint at C5-6 (*white arrow* in [A]).

claimed that he had been suspended in revenge for having testified as an expert witness for the plaintiff in a medical malpractice suit brought against another member of the association. The court noted that Dr Austin, by testifying at trial, provided a type of medical service and was subject to peer review by professional associations and further cited the Health Care Quality Improvement Act of 1986 (HCQIA) as giving relative immunity to peer review organizations. Although there is some prospect for emending the flaws in the system through this means, the matter is essentially not yet settled. In 2006, a Florida court parsed the words of the HCQIA, noting that peer-review immunity granted by the act related to direct patient care and not to testimony given in court.[60] Thus, other professional societies, such as the College of American Pathologies, chose not to pursue expert witness peer review for fear of being sued.[61]

SUMMARY

One of the major pitfalls faced by physicians is a basic lack of understanding of the legal aspects of medical malpractice. It is the authors' hope that the brief review of the history of malpractice law provided here will afford the radiologist insights that could prove helpful in understanding how one must conduct oneself in a radiology practice. There are several noteworthy points to consider. Vigilance and minimizing errors is always most desirable, but error-free neuroradiology is unattainable. Best medical judgment, although not error free, is at least defensible as noted in the case law discussed here. Errors of protocol, on the other hand, are extremely difficult to defend, particular failure to communicate significant results. Understanding this alone will reduce risk immeasurably. Errors resulting from bias, particularly alliterative errors, are most insidious and require significant self-vigilance. It should be noted that many of these errors, as well as perceptual errors, are the result of rushing, distraction, or fatigue resulting from excessive workloads. Errors, such as missing the corner finding, are not discussed here but are also common errors leading to litigation whose source also lies in carelessness or fatigue. Other pitfalls are not under the radiologist's control; one unfortunately cannot easily choose the clinical colleagues associated with his or her practice but vigilance for their errors can certainly reduce the risk of being sued. Finally, because postoperative neuroimaging studies and C-spine trauma are both so commonly performed and so commonly associated with malpractice litigation, heightened caution and vigilance for the difficult pathologic conditions discussed here will also help one bypass avoidable liability.

REFERENCES

1. Epstein NE. It is easier to confuse a jury than convince a judge: the crisis in medical malpractice. Spine 2002;27:2425–30.
2. Berlin L. Radiologic malpractice litigation: a view of the past, a gaze at the present, a glimpse of the future. AJR Am J Roentgenol 2003;181:1481–6.
3. Good reads. James Madison quotes. Available at: http://www.goodreads.com/author/quotes/63859. James_Madison. Accessed June 26, 2012.
4. Medical malpractice insurance costs and coverage. New York: Greater New York Hospital Association; 2005.
5. AANS. Study analyzes how the malpractice environment impacts practicing neurosurgeons. Medical News Today. MediLexicon Intl; 2008. Available at: http://www.medicalnewstoday.com/releases/105599. php. Accessed January 28, 2012.
6. Mohajer ST. California regulator: malpractice insurance too pricey. The Associated Press; 2011.
7. The Economist. Scalpel, scissors, lawyer. London: Form Copyright The Economist Newspaper Ltd; 2005.
8. Reynolds RA, Rizzo JA, Gonzalez ML. The cost of medical professional liability. JAMA 1987;257:2776–81.
9. Mello M, Chandra A, Gawande AA, et al. National costs of the medical liability system. Health Aff 2009;29(9):1569–77.
10. Jena AB, Seabury S, Lakdawalla D, et al. Malpractice risk according to physician specialty. N Engl J Med 2011;365:629–36.
11. Dick JF 3rd, Gallagher TH, Brenner RJ, et al. Predictors of radiologists' perceived risk of malpractice lawsuits in breast imaging. Am J Roentgenol 2009; 192(2):327–33.
12. Baker SR, Harkisoon S. The causes of malpractice suits in radiology: the contemporary records of 5300 radiologists. In: RSNA scientific posters: Radiological Society of North America Scientific Assembly and Annual Meeting Program. Chicago: Radiological Society of North America; 2004. p. 554.
13. Physician Insurers Association of America - PIAA – 2005.
14. Sanbar SS, Firestone MH. Medical malpractice stress syndrome. In: Sanbar SS, editor. Medical malpractice survival handbook. Philadelphia: American College of Legal Medicine, Elsevier Inc; 2007.
15. Blackstone W. Commentaries on the laws of England. Oxford (England): Clarendon; 1768. p. 122.
16. Cross V Guthrey, 2 Root 90, Conn (1794).
17. Rosenbaum S. Law and the public's health: medical errors, medical negligence, and professional medical liability reform. Public Health Rep 2003;118:272–4.
18. Landon V. Humphrey, 9 Conn 209, 1832.
19. McCandless V. McWha, 22 Pa 261, 1853.
20. MacKinzie V. Carman, 92 NYS 1063–1067 (1905).
21. Department of Regulation and Licensing v State of Wisconsin Medical Examining Board, 572 NW2d 508 (Wis App 1997).
22. Siegle RL, Baram EM, Reuter SR, et al. Rates of disagreement in imaging interpretation in a group of community hospitals. Acad Radiol 1998;5:148–54.
23. Lehr JL, Lodwick GS, Farrell C, et al. Direct measurement of the effect of film miniaturization on diagnostic accuracy. Radiology 1976;118:257–63.
24. Berlin L. Does the "missed" radiographic diagnosis constitute malpractice? Radiology 1977;123:523–7.
25. Berlin L, Hendrix RW. Perceptual errors and negligence. Am J Roentgenol 1998;170:863–7.
26. Berlin L. Communication of the significant but not urgent finding. Am J Roentgenol 1997;168:329–31.

27. Berlin L. Failure of radiologic communication: an increasing cause of malpractice litigation and harm to patients. Appl Radiol 2010;39:17–23.

28. American College of Radiology. ACR standard for communication: diagnostic radiology. In: Standards. Reston (VA): American College of Radiology; 1997. p. 5–6.

29. Williams V. Le, 662 SE2d 73 (Va 2008).

30. Betesh V. United States of America, 400 F Supp 238 (US Dist DC 1974).

31. Daly V. United States of America, 946 F2d, 1467 (9th Cir 1991).

32. Stanley V. McCarver, 92 P3d 849 (Ariz 2004).

33. Raskin MM. Survival strategies for radiology: Some practical tips on how to reduce the risk of being sued and losing. J Am Coll Radiol 2006;3:689–93.

34. Aideyan UO, Berbaum K, Smith WL. Influence of prior radiologic information on the interpretation of radiographic examinations. Acad Radiol 1995;2:205–8.

35. Doubilet P, Herman PG. Interpretation of radiographs: effect of clinical history. AJR Am J Roentgenol 1981;137:1055–8.

36. Elmore JG, Wells CK, Howard DH, et al. The impact of clinical history on mammographic interpretations. JAMA 1997;227:49–52.

37. Smith MJ. Error and variation in diagnostic radiology. Springfield (IL): Thomas; 1967. p. 75–7.

38. Berlin L. Malpractice issues in radiology: alliterative errors. Am J Roentgenol 2000;174:925–30.

39. Hlavin ML, Kaminski HJ, Fenstermaker RA, et al. Intracranial suppuration: a modern decade of postoperative subdural empyema and epidural abscess. Neurosurgery 1994;34:974–81.

40. Lekovic GP, Harrington TR. Litigation of missed cervical spine injuries in patients presenting with blunt traumatic injury. Neurosurgery 2007;60(3):516–23.

41. American College of Radiology (2009). ACR appropriateness criteria: suspected spine trauma. Available at: http://www.acr.org/SecondaryMainMenuCategories/quality_safety/app_criteria/pdf/ExpertPanelon MusculoskeletalImaging/SuspectedCervicalSpine TraumaDoc22.asp. Accessed June 25, 2012. American College of Radiology. ACR practice guideline for communication of diagnostic imaging findings. Revised 2010 (Resolution 11).

42. Schoenfeld AJ, Bono CM, McGuire KJ, et al. Computed tomography alone versus computed tomography and magnetic resonance imaging in the identification of occult injuries to the cervical spine: a meta-analysis. J Trauma 2010;68(1):109–13.

43. Schuster R, Waxman K, Sanchez B, et al. Magnetic resonance imaging is not needed to clear cervical spines in blunt trauma patients with normal computed tomographic results and no motor deficits. Arch Surg 2005;140(8):762–6.

44. Tomycz ND, Chew BG, Chang YF, et al. MRI is unnecessary to clear the cervical spine in obtunded/comatose trauma patients: the four-year experience of a level I trauma center. J Trauma 2008;64(5):1258–63.

45. Kallmes DF, Layton K, Marx WF, et al. Death by nondiagnosis: why emergent CT angiography should not be done for patients with subarachnoid hemorrhage. AJNR Am J Neuroradiol 2007;28(10): 1837–8.

46. Fox AJ, Symons SP, Aviv RI. CT angiography is state-of-the-art first vascular imaging for subarachnoid hemorrhage. AJNR Am J Neuroradiol 2008; 29(6):e41–2.

47. Gold R, Reichman M, Greenberg E, et al. Developing a new reference standard: is validation necessary? Acad Radiol 2010;17(9):1079–82.

48. Cheah TS. The impact of clinical guidelines and clinical pathways on medical practice: effectiveness and medico-legal aspects. Ann Acad Med Singap 1998;27(4):533–9.

49. Papke K, Brassel F. Modern cross-sectional imaging in the diagnosis and follow-up of intracranial aneurysms. Eur Radiol 2006;16(9):2051–66.

50. Adams WM, Laitt RD, Jackson A. The role of MR angiography in the pretreatment assessment of intracranial aneurysms: a comparative study. AJNR Am J Neuroradiol 2000;21(9):1618–28.

51. Li Q, Lv F, Li Y, et al. Evaluation of 64-section CT angiography for detection and treatment planning of intracranial aneurysms by using DSA and surgical findings. Radiology 2009;252(3):808–15.

52. Kim PE, Fassihi A, Go JL, et al. Another approach to determining sensitivity of CT angiography for detection of cerebral aneurysms. Presented at the American Society of Neuroradiology, 43rd Annual Meeting. Toronto, Ontario, Canada, May 21–27, 2005.

53. Villablanca JP, Jahan R, Hooshi P, et al. Detection and characterization of very small cerebral aneurysms by using 2D and 3D helical CT angiography. AJNR Am J Neuroradiol 2002;23(7):1187–98.

54. Menke J, Larsen J, Kallenberg K. Diagnosing cerebral aneurysms by computed tomographic angiography: meta-analysis. Ann Neurol 2011; 69(4):646–54.

55. Jayaraman MV, Mayo-Smith WW, Tung GA, et al. Detection of intracranial aneurysms: multi-detector row CT angiography compared with DSA. Radiology 2004;230(2):510–8.

56. Byun CK, Go JL, Lerner A, et al. Decreased accuracy of CT angiography for small intracranial aneurysms compared to DSA is operator dependent and not an inherent characteristic of CT angiography. Presented at the American Society of Neuroradiology, 49th Annual Meeting, Seattle (WA), June 4–9, 2011.

57. Provenzale JM, Kranz PG. Dural sinus thrombosis: sources of error in image interpretation. AJR Am J Roentgenol 2011;196(1):23–31.

58. Austin V. American Association of Neurological Surgeons, 253 F. 3d 967 (7th Cir. 2001).

59. Thompson TL. ACR expels member for improper lawsuit testimony. Radiology News, Auntminnie.com, July 9, 2004. Available at: http://www.auntminnie.com/index.aspx?sec=sup&sub=imc&pag=dis&ItemID=62257. Accessed June 25, 2012.

60. Fullerton V. Florida Medical Association, Inc., 938 So. 2d 587 (Fla. Dist Ct, App. 2006).

61. Finkel E. Clash act: peer review of expert witness testimony. Feature Story, CAP Today, October 2006. Available at: http://www.cap.org/apps/cap.portal?_nfpb=true&cntvwrPtlt_actionOverride=%2Fportlets%2FcontentViewer%2Fshow&_windowLabel=cntvwrPtlt&cntvwrPtlt%7BactionForm.contentReference%7D=cap_today%2Ffeature_stories%2F1006ExpertWit.html&_state=maximized&_pageLabel=cntvwr. Accessed June 25, 2012.

Index

Note: Page numbers of article titles are in **boldface** type.

Neuroimag Clin N Am 22 (2012) 539–542
http://dx.doi.org/10.1016/S1052-5149(12)00096-2
1052-5149/12/$ – see front matter © 2012 Elsevier Inc. All rights reserved

neuroimaging.theclinics.com